Blueprint for Holistic Healing

Blueprint for Holistic Healing

Your Practical Guide to Body-Mind-Spirit Health

C. Norman Shealy, MD, PhD

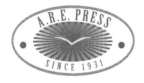

A.R.E. Press • Virginia Beach • Virginia

A.R.E. Press
215 67th Street
Virginia Beach, VA 23451-2061

ISBN 13: 978-0-87604-809-2

Disclaimer

The material in this book is not intended to replace conventional medical advice. You should consult your physician regarding any general or specific physical symptoms. The author and publisher disclaim any responsibility for adverse effects resulting from information in this book.

During Edgar Cayce's life, the Edgar Cayce readings were all numbered to provide confidentiality. So in the case of 294-1, for example, the first set of numbers ("294") refers to the individual or group for whom the reading was given. The second set of numbers ("1") refers to the number in the series from which the reading is taken. Therefore, 294-1 identifies the reading as the first one given to the individual assigned #294.

Cover design by Christine Fulcher

Contents

Overview

Body—physical, chemical, emotional, metaphysical

Mind—personality, mood, attitudes and emotions, beliefs, cultural, social, ethnic

Soul vs. Spirit

DO IT NOW

There is no meaning unless you make it.
There is no step unless YOU take it.
Not one goal you can't achieve–
But first you must roll up that sleeve . . .

Always has been graft and greed
Don't let that stop you.

You can be freed—

Be the exception
No matter how
Make the meaning.
Do it NOW.

Georgianne Ginder
2006

Acknowledgments

Although I grew up "knowing" that I was more than my body and mind and never doubted that there was another "me" that somehow existed in an ineffable time/space, the real understanding of myself as an entity separate from my body took place in 1972 during my first visit to the A.R.E. when I had my first out–of–body experience. To the entire Edgar Cayce work and Association and to Joel Andrews, the trance medium harpist, I owe the sense of being beyond body and mind. Indeed, although my intuition has always been active, I believe that that one event opened me to many developing psychic events. Thank you! And thanks especially to Kevin Todeschi for suggesting I write this book!

Of course my parents were responsible for outstanding nurturing and encouragement to explore the world.

My wife, Mary–Charlotte Bayles Shealy, provided fifty–two blessed years of total support for thinking outside the box of conventional society, as well as the foundation for grounding our children in the same expansion of consciousness that is so essential to real life.

Henry Rucker, Robert Leichtman, MD, and Caroline Myss have been the most outstanding intuitives I have known. They have further nurtured my ongoing curiosity about the physical and spiritual worlds.

I have also been remarkably blessed by numerous outstanding teachers, friends, and associates. Having "known" many of my past lives, several of which I am not proud, it is again the A.R.E. where I had my first past–life experience. These continue to amaze me, especially reconnection with the reincarnated St. Francis and my three brothers/companions from our lives with Francis. These have provided the most remarkable living love of my ongoing life. Thank you Peter, Mark, Patrick, and Sergey!

I am grateful to Georgie Ginder for contributing the wonderful poem you have just read.

To all who read this book, I wish for you the bliss of **knowing yourself** in the broadest possible way—physically, mentally, emotionally and spiritually!

Love and **hugs**,
Norm

1 Holism

The whole is greater than the sum of the parts. Basically, it is virtually impossible to discuss body, mind, and spirit as individual entities, as they are intricately interwoven and interdependent. Mind is the builder and body is the result. It is the soul incarnate that provides human life. Spirit is the connection of soul with the divine or God. In medicine, René Descartes is credited with the scientific separation of body, mind, and soul. He felt that the body is materially present in a physical sense and that the mind is essentially immaterial—it has no physical manifestations. To a great extent this is the philosophy of science and of modern medicine.

In 1929 Jan Smuts, general and prime minister of South Africa, introduced the word *holism* in a masterpiece book, *Holism and Evolution.* From early 1900 until 1945, Edgar Cayce laid the foundation for the remarkably broad field of holistic medicine. I was introduced to the Cayce material in 1972, and it changed my life forever, awakening my interest in all aspects of health and mysticism. In 1978, with the founding of the American Holistic Medical Association, www.holisticmedicine.org, I envisioned that at least 10% of physicians would become holistically inclined within ten years. Actually, the number of out-of-the-closet holistic physicians has changed little through the ensuing thirty-six years, but it has been the main source for truly holistic medicine! Despite having the American Board of Holistic Medicine, AHMA membership has not kept up with the actual growth in total physicians. Now, to my surprise, the current leadership of AHMA has decided that the word *holistic* will never be accepted by the Establishment and voted to drop holistic in favor of integrated—a word already highly polluted by hospitals *pretending* to be inclusive. The Establishment is the problem, not the solution!

Most physicians are too brainwashed by the PharmacoMafia and remain sheepishly oblivious to the broader human perspective. In 1978, I was excited at the need for holistic medicine. Initially, my sense of great need was the result of being appalled by the barbarian approaches to chronic pain—cordotomy, cutting the front half of the spinal cord, and frontal lobotomy, destroying the personality forever. In 1971, having introduced Transcutaneous Electrical Nerve Stimulation (TENS) and Dorsal Column Stimulation (DCS), I was overwhelmed with four hundred patients each year. I selected only 6% at most for the DCS and most of the rest were much too complex for TENS. Almost all were iatrogenically addicted to Valium® and Percodan®. They had had an average of five to seven unsuccessful surgeries; they had an average of forty-nine symptoms. Clearly the system had failed them.

Between 1971 and 1978, I added acupuncture, biofeedback, past-life therapy, music therapy, massage and exercise, nutrition, and gradually a wide variety of self-regulation techniques. I sensed the broad **spiritual crisis** that many patients had endured. Thus was the need for a return to spiritual healing at all levels. I naively thought that we would have several thousand physicians join the holistic movement within a few years. The AMA rejected the concept from the beginning. Then a few hospitals paid lip service and started mentioning the very word. However, the *practice* of comprehensive holism never took hold and soon the acceptable terms became complementary and alternative. Finally, the current **pretend** is integrative medicine, with many hospitals paying slightly more than lip service and offering a few alternatives—**never holistic or comprehensive**.

Meanwhile, the broadest scientific field of all, energy medicine, evolved to include everything outside drugs and surgery. Holism began to be relegated to the past. Even the American Holistic Medical Association voted to drop the word holistic, because the current leaders believe the term would never be accepted by the Establishment. Of course it is the Establishment, which is more constipated and fixed on ignoring the basic *cause* of disease—**stress**! At least a huge majority of disease is the result of **spiritual distress**, leading to anxiety and depression and ultimately to a majority of illnesses!

If the *cause* is spiritual, the solution must be **holistic**—the basic meaning of which is *holy*. This spiritual **existential** crisis leads to hopelessness, poor self-esteem, and failure to take care of *self*. Ultimately it is recognition that the body is the temple of the soul, which requires attention to the *self*—mind, spirit, and soul working together to heal the body and to keep it healthy.

Practicing in a comprehensive holistic clinic between 1971 and 2003, I worked with over 30,000 patients who had been failed by conventional medicine. For three years our clinic was named by the American Academy of Pain Management as the most cost effective and the most successful for management of chronic pain. Our success rate was consistently 85%. Of course virtually all the patients had depression as well as a wide variety of medical problems in addition to pain.

I tried for twenty years to find a holistic physician to take over the clinic. Failing that, I closed the clinic in 2003 and have focused on research and writing. Almost daily I receive requests to see difficult patients who have been failed by the system. I am asked many times a week for referral to a holistic physician. There are about a thousand who are members of the devolving AHMA, but I know of no truly comprehensive clinic. There are, of course, a few excellent clinics which offer some great alternatives.

With the advent of the Unaffordable Care Act, it is estimated that 30% of physicians will retire early and the system may well collapse, while offering, at best, drugs and surgery—critical perhaps 15% of the time and failing almost always even to acknowledge the underlying spiritual crisis. Even with our system already costing over twice that of any other western country, the US remains about number 37 on the totem pole of health. The only *hope* is a turn to holism!

In the 90s Congress "mandated" at NIH a National Center for Complementary and Alternative Medicine(NCCAM), which funds some research but rather a paltry amount compared to mainstream PharmacoMafia work. Indeed, the vast majority of American physicians and medical journals are today pawns of the PharmacoMafia! Silently almost half of physicians personally use some Complementary and Alternative Medicine (CAM) approaches but only about 16% admit to ever referring a patient for such safe alternatives. Despite the negligence of physicians in truthfully evaluating and using many of the safe alternative approaches to health, the American public has embraced the field to the extent that more than 50% of Americans use some "nonmedical" alternative approach every year. Indeed, I believe unequivocally that at least 85% of illnesses should be treated comprehensively with these safer and more effective alternatives. There is a need for conventional medicine—mostly in acute illnesses and injuries. On the other hand, if individuals take responsibility for their lifestyle and live a healthy life, most illnesses can be avoided.

Almost twenty years ago Dr. Elmer Green, father of biofeedback, organized the International Society for the Study of Subtle Energy and Energy Medicine, www.issseem.org. Thus energy medicine became another of the new terms.

Hospitals have most often jumped belatedly into the marketplace offering their form of integrative medicine, which means that they espouse integrating some alternatives. Most often they do a crappy job and prostitute the whole concept.

The CAM approaches recognized by the NCCAM are:
1. Nutrition and Lifestyle: diet, exercise, sleep, and stress management
2. Mind–Body Medicine
3. Alternative systems of Medical Thought: Traditional Chinese Medicine
4. Alternative systems of Medical Thought: Yoga and Ayurveda
5. Alternative systems of Medical Thought: Homeopathy
6. Bioenergetic Medicine
7. Pharmacologic/Biologically based: Herbal Medicine
8. Pharmacologic/Biologically based: nutrition, dietary supplements, and vitamins

9. Manipulative Therapies: Chiropractic, Osteopathic

10. Manipulative Therapies: Massage

The American Student Medical Association (ASMA) established sylla-bi for teaching all these CAM approaches, but few medical schools offer anything significant in these fields. To a great extent all of these fields can just as easily be considered holistic medicine, integrative medi-cine, or energy medicine. Of course, I have to mention that spiritual and soul medicines are part of mind–body medicine and are the most critical issues avoided by the Establishment and integrative medicine. I am pleased to have written the ASMA syllabus for training in mind-body medicine. *Conventional* American medicine uses only drugs and surgery—none of the more critical issues are addressed by most MDs and DOs.

My own practice began in 1971 to offer all the CAM categories. The Shealy Institute and Shealy Wellness Center became the most cost-ef-fective and most patient–effective clinic I know. Ninety–plus percent of what we did required no physician. That is why I founded Holos Uni-versity Graduate Seminar, www.holosuniversity.org, to train competent individuals in the broad field of spiritual healing and energy medicine. These include essentially all the CAM, holistic, integrative, and energy medicine approaches to health.

In 2008, my movie, *Medical Renaissance—The Secret Code*, www.Medical-Renaissance.net, was produced. It is the best overall presentation I know to demonstrate the effectiveness of holistic medicine. Recently I have released the most exciting result of the influence of spiritual intuition—rejuvenation of DNA telomeres, the key to life, health, and longevity! For the first time in history, we have demonstrated rejuvenation and regrowth of this key to health and longevity!

As mentioned before, I receive almost daily requests for referrals to a truly holistic clinic. The only way I can see a solution to this problem is to begin again and to create the model for holism, the International Institute of Holistic Medicine, which has now been done with a world-class migraine specialist, a world–class cardiologist, a world–class sound physician, and the original pain and depression specialist in Springfield, Missouri.

This book explores the many dimensions needed to integrate body, mind, and soul into the holistic whole. In 1988 Caroline Myss and I co-authored *The Creation of Health*, in which she wrote the metaphysical intuitive concepts of health and disease while I dealt with the medical concepts. Here, I hope to integrate an even broader overview of life itself.

In the late 70s, Dr. John Knowles wrote a hallmark article, *The Responsibility of the Individual*. He stated, "99% of individuals are born healthy and become unhealthy because of human misbehavior." Today statistics state that only 95% of babies are born healthy and a striking 12% nationally are born prematurely! Forty percent of babies are born to single mothers, setting the stage for the greatest possible variety of the ideal, because inviting a soul to incarnate requires two potential parents who love one another and carefully prepare fully for the possibility of a healthy child who will be nurtured to optimal life.

If both parents are truly healthy and reasonably well-adjusted mentally and share spiritual ideals, then the soul choosing to incarnate with them has the best potential to arrive physically healthy. Obviously there are rare genetic inheritances that may show up despite the best of plans. Nevertheless, with this foundation the chances are at least 99% that the baby will be born healthy.

The requirements for such ideal parents are between the ages of 25 and 35, socially well-adjusted with adequate income. They do not smoke and they drink alcohol moderately, if at all. They have a body mass index of 18 to 24. They eat at least five total servings daily of fruits and vegetables. They exercise a minimum of thirty minutes at least five days a week. Unfortunately, only 3% of Americans have these essential basic habits! In addition to these critical habits, this couple will likely take some supplements, perhaps at least Vitamin D 3, a minimum of 2000 units daily and a multivitamin-mineral with up to 25 mg of B complex, with a minimum of 1000 mcg of folic acid, and at least 1000 unit of Omega-3s. During the pregnancy, the couple will avoid significant stresses, such as fluoridated, chlorinated water; smog, and excessive exposure to electromagnetic pollution. They will have regular spiritual practices, setting the mental and emotional stage for a nurturing welcome to the baby. Although I will attempt to deal with possible corrective measures for some health problems, I prefer to start with the ideals for an optimally healthy baby and childhood first.

The parents will avoid today's Round-Up® polluted wheat and the vast majority of packaged foods, as well as *all* "fast food" restaurants, sugar, monosodium glutamate, hydrogenated fats, all artificial sweeteners, substitutes, and artificial additives.

At the end of nine months the mother will go into labor and have a reasonably comfortable delivery, without anesthesia or significant drugs. The healthy baby will be welcomed and kept with the mother, who will nurse it for at least the first six months of life.

Statistically, if this baby has good health habits, it will live an average of one hundred years. If it adopts the average American habits, it will live only seventy-eight years. The difference in longevity is likely to involve many more problems. Life in the US is shortened by accidents, stokes, heart attacks, cancer, infections, and a wide variety of problems—most of which are the results of behaviors and habits.

Smoking shortens life by an average of six to seven years for each pack of cigarettes smoked daily. Obesity shortens life as much as smoking three packs daily, if the person is forty or more pounds overweight. Unfortunately, being a man shortens life by about three years over that of a woman's.

Excellent studies have shown that the major causes of premature death are:

- Obesity
- Smoking
- Medical services
- Poor nutrition
- Inactivity
- Inadequate sleep

Only three percent of Americans have the essentials:

- normal body weight
- no smoking
- adequate intake, five servings daily, of fruits and vegetables
- exercise of thirty minutes five days a week!

If all Americans had these habits, within twenty-five years, average American life would be one hundred instead of the current seventy-eight. Therefore, to start our discussion of a healthy body, it is critical to emphasize that true health is virtually impossible without these habits. Indeed, with these habits our major diseases of heart attack, hypertension, stroke, and cancer would be diminished 75 to 80%! Essentially, a vast majority of illness and premature death results from not caring for self. And this care-*less*-ness appears to be the result of low self-esteem, depression, and anxiety. Thus, I begin with evaluating the stress that is the foundation of a huge majority of disease.

2 Stress and Distress

Sixty years ago in medical school, I was told that 75% of all the patients I would see would be there because of stress. **But** not one word was said about treating that stress! Indeed, even the major cascade of stress was not significantly taught. In the late 70s Joseph Califano, Secretary of HEW, emphasized that the only way we would decrease disease was to **prevent it**. But there has been minimal attention to preventing disease. And shortly after Califano's statement, Dr. John Knowles wrote that "Ninety-nine percent of people are born healthy and become unhealthy because of human misbehavior." The human misbehavior that Knowles was emphasizing was the responsibility of the individual. I will emphasize also the misbehavior of society in the broader sense, as well as the individual!

In order to understand personal responsibilities, I start with emotions, as they provide the foundation for the stressors that most people know and consider the "cause" of their distress. Basically, there is only one major emotional stress—*fear*. And there are only five significant fears:
- Death

- Invalidism
- Poverty
- Abandonment—loss of love
- Existential issues—purpose, meaning, why, justice, and God

Our reactions to *fear* are:

- Anxiety
- Anger
- Guilt
- Depression
- And dozens of synonyms for each of these!

All of these are associated with a remarkable cascade of chemical reactions which result in mental, emotional, and physical stress. The basic chemical reaction is the release of adrenalin, which raises blood pressure and pulse, and leads to the release of cortisol and sugar, which leads to the release of insulin and DHEA, dehydroepiandrosterone, to help bring down the blood cortisol. Incidentally, blood cholesterol is increased by virtually all stressors. This basic reaction may result from mental experiences of anxiety, anger, guilt, or depression *or* the stress response may be induced by:

- Caffeine
- Tobacco/nicotine
- Sugar
- Alcohol
- Inadequate oxygen
- Excess carbon dioxide
- Excess heat or cold
- Inactivity
- Physical pressures/injuries
- Toxins, of which there are a few "natural" and over 550,000 human-made ones
- Nuclear energy/radiation

Essentially, a stress response is one which **doubles** the blood level of adrenalin or epinephrine. Simple examples in one not previously exposed:

- One cigarette
- One cup of coffee
- 8 ounces of "pop"
- 5 teaspoons of sugar
- One ounce of alcohol, one beer, or one glass of wine

• Being totally inactive

The great stress researcher, Hans Selye, emphasized the fact that we accommodate to repeated stress, so that with the same small stress, within a short period of time, perhaps a week of daily exposure, minimal adrenalin is released. *But every time we adapt to a stressor, we decrease our tolerance to new stressors.* Thus, we begin the process of maladaptation, which leads to virtually every known disease, degeneration, exhaustion, and death. Stress is thus additive or cumulative. Our genetic inheritance and our social environment are also inherent foundations upon which our stress reactions occur. And, of course, I believe that most genetic influences are significantly present because of karmic unfinished business. In other words, all significant illnesses are the result of unfinished psychological problems from a previous life!

Thus a baby born healthy and lovingly nurtured has far more resistance to unavoidable stressors than one born unhealthy. In the healthy situation, assuming reasonably good nutrition and moderate physical activity, a child continues to be healthy into young adulthood. Beginning at puberty, one of the most important hormonal regulators of stress, DHEA, begins to increase and reaches a peak production at age 25. Adolescent jocks may reach that peak in the mid-teens, emphasizing the additional benefits of increased physical exercise. By age 25 the healthy male has a blood level of DHEA between 750 and 1250 nanograms per deciliter. A healthy female has blood levels of 500 to 980 nanograms per deciliter. By age 30 the average person has lost 10% of his DHEA and by age 80 the average person has lost 80 to 90% of his peak DHEA. Thus, the simplest measurement of stress reserves is a blood test of free DHEA. The only lab I trust for this critical hormone test is Nichols in Capistrano, California. I have no financial interest in the lab, but extensive research has shown that five major labs give results that are 50 to 300% different on the same blood. *Most DHEA is attached to a sulfur molecule and DHEA-S is not a reliable test of DHEA availability! Actually DHEA deficiency is only the tip of the iceberg of adrenal fatigue, which I will address later.*

Cumulative **total life stress** is the reason for the gradually declining DHEA levels and the slow maladaptation that leads to virtually all illnesses, other than some accidents. Here is an excellent time to evaluate your Total Life Stress. One point represents essentially a doubling of cortisone or adrenalin output in response to the stressor:

PERSONAL STRESS ASSESSMENT
Total Life Stress Test

NAME _____ DATE _____

Record your stress points on the lines in the right-hand margin, and indicate subtotals in the boxes at the end of each section. Then add your subtotals (on page 135) to determine your total score.

A. DIETARY STRESS
Average Daily Sugar Consumption

Sugar added to food or drink	1 point per 5 teaspoons	___
Sweet roll, piece of pie/cake, brownie, other dessert	1 point each	___
Coke or can of pop; candy bar	2 points each	___
Banana split, commercial milk shake, sundae, etc.	5 points each	___
White flour (white bread, spaghetti, etc.)	5 points	___

Average Daily Salt Consumption

Little or no "added" salt	0 points	___
Few salty foods (pretzels, potato chips, etc.)	0 points	___
Moderate "added" salt and/or salty foods at least once per day	3 points	___
Heavy salt user, regularly (use of "table salt" and/or salty foods at least twice per day)	10 points	___

Average Daily Caffeine Consumption

Coffee	½ point each cup	___
Tea	½ point each cup	___
Cola drink or Mountain Dew	1 point each cup	___
2 Anacin or APC tabs	½ point per dose	___
Caffeine Benzoate tablets (NoDoz, Vivarin, etc.)	2 points each	___

Average Weekly Eating Out

2-4 times per week	3 points	___
5-10 times per week	6 points	___
More than 10 times per week	10 points	___

DIETARY SUBTOTAL [   ] A

B. ENVIRONMENTAL STRESS
Drinking Water
Chlorinated only	1 point	____
Chlorinated and fluoridated	2 points	____

Soil and Air Pollution
Live within 10 miles of city of 500,000 or more	10 points	____
Live within 10 miles of city of 250,000 or more	5 points	____
Live within 10 miles of city of 50,000 or more	2 points	____
Live in the country but use pesticides, herbicides, and/or chemical fertilizer	10 points	____
Exposed to cigarette smoke of someone else more than 1 hour per day	5 points	____

Television Watched
For each hour over 1 per day	½ point	____
	ENVIRONMENTAL	[ ] B

C. CHEMICAL STRESS
Drugs (any amount of usage)
Antidepressants	1 point	____
Tranquilizers	3 points	____
Sleeping pills	3 points	____
Narcotics	5 points	____
Other pain relievers	3 points	____

Nicotine
3-10 cigarettes per day	5 points	____
11-20 cigarettes per day	15 points	____
21-30 cigarettes per day	20 points	____
31-40 cigarettes per day	35 points	____
Over 40 cigarettes per day	40 points	____
Cigar(s) per day	1 point each	____
Pipeful(s) of tobacco per day	1 point each	____
Chewing tobacco -"chews" per day	1 point each	____

Average Daily Alcohol Consumption
1 oz. whiskey, gin, vodka, etc.	2 points each	____
8 oz. beer	2 points each	____
4-6 oz. glass of wine	2 points each	____
	CHEMICAL SUBTOTAL	[ ] C

D. PHYSICAL STRESS
Weight

Underweight more than 10 lbs.	5 points	____
10 to 15 lbs. overweight	5 points	____
16 to 25 lbs. overweight	10 points	____
26 to 40 lbs. overweight	25 points	____
More than 40 lbs. overweight	40 points	____

Activity

Adequate exercise*, 3 days or more per week	0 points	____
Some physical exercise, 1 or 2 days per week	15 points	____
No regular exercise	40 points	____

Work Stress

Sit most of the day	3 points	____
Industrial/factory worker	3 points	____
Overnight travel more than once a week	5 points	____
Work more than 50 hours per week	2 points per hour over 50	____
Work night shift	5 points	____

PHYSICAL SUBTOTAL [   ] D

*Adequate means doubling heartbeat and/or sweating minimum of 30 minutes per time.

E. Holmes-Rahe Social Readjustment Rating*

(Circle the mean values that correspond with life events listed below which you have experienced during the past 12 months.)

Death of spouse	100
Divorce	73
Marital separation	65
Jail term	63
Death of close family member	63
Personal injury or illness	53
Marriage	50
Fired at work	47
Marital reconciliation	45
Retirement	45
Change in health of family member	44
Pregnancy	40
Sexual difficulties	39
Gain of new family member	39
Business readjustment	39
Change in financial state	38
Death of close friend	37
Change to different line of work	36
Change in number of arguments with spouse	35
Mortgage over $20,000	31
Foreclosure of mortgage or loan	30
Change in responsibilities at work	29
Son or daughter leaving home	29
Trouble with in-laws	29
Outstanding personal achievement	28
Spouse begins or stops work	26
Begin or end school	25
Change in living conditions	24
Revision of personal habits	23
Trouble with boss	20

Change in work hours or conditions	20
Change in residence	20
Change in schools	19
Change in recreation	19
Change in church activities	18
Change in social activities	17
Mortgage or loan less than $20,000	16
Change in sleeping habits	15
Change in eating habits	15
Vacation, especially if away from home	13
Christmas or other major holiday stress	12
Minor violations of the law	11

(Add the mean values to get the Holmes-Rahe total. Then refer to the conversion table to determine your number of points.)

Conversion Table

Holmes-Rahe less than	60	110	160	170	180	190	200	210	220	230	240	250	260	265	270	275	280	285	290	295	300	305	310	315	320	325	330	335	340	345	350	Anything over 351=40+
Your number of points:	0	1	2	3	4	5	6	7	8	9	10	11	12	13	14	15	16	17	18	19	20	21	22	23	24	25	26	27	28	29	30	

Holmes-Rahe Social Readjustment Rating (Converted) [   ] E

*The Social Readjustment Rating Scale: See Holmes. T. H. and Rahe, R.H.: The social readjustment raring scale. *Journal of Psychosomatic Research.* 11:213218, 1967, for complete wording; of these items. Reproduced with permission of the authors and publisher.

EMOTIONAL STRESS

Sleep

Less than 7 hours per night	3 points	___
Usually 7 or 8 hours per night	0 points	___
More than 8 hours per night	2 points	___

Relaxation

Relax only during sleep	10 points	___
Relax or meditate at least 20 minutes per day	0 points	___

Frustration at Work

Enjoy work	0 points	___
Mildly frustrated by job	1 point	___
Moderately frustrated by job	3 points	___
Very frustrated by job	5 points	___

Marital Status

Married, happily	0 points	___
Married, moderately unhappy	2 points	___
Married, very unhappy	5 points	___
Unmarried man over 30	5 points	___
Unmarried woman over 30	2 points	___

Usual Mood

Happy, well adjusted	0 points	___
Moderately angry, depressed, or frustrated	10 points	___
Very angry, depressed, or frustrated	20 points	___

Any Other Major Stress Not Mentioned Above—
You Judge Intensity (Specify):
_____ (10 to 40 points)

EMOTIONAL
SUBTOTAL [   ] F

Add A _____ +B _____ +C _____

+D+E _____ +F _____   _____

YOUR PERSONAL STRESS ASSESSMENT SCORE

If your score exceeds 25 points, you probably will feel better if you reduce your stress; greater than 50 points, you definitely need to eliminate stress in your life.

Circle your stressor with the highest number of points and work first to eliminate it; then circle your next greatest stressor, overcome it; and so on.

SELF-HEALTH SYSTEMS OF BRINDABELLA FARMS
5607 South 222nd Rd. • Fair Grove, Missouri 65648
Phone: 417-267-2900 • Fax: 417-267-3102

The higher your Total Life Stress, the higher the number of symptoms.

SYMPTOM INDEX

Name: _____ Date: _____

When people are chronically ill, they often have other symptoms. Do you have any of the following? *Please check only those that you have now or recently.*

____ Depressed mood
____ Loss of interest or pleasure in things you used to enjoy
____ Significant weight change (loss or gain)
____ Frequent eating between meals
____ Insomnia
____ Snoring
____ Sleepwalking
____ Hypersomnia
____ Agitation
____ Sluggishness, slow to function
____ Fatigue, low energy, or feeling tired all of the time
____ Feelings of worthlessness or guilt
____ Difficulty concentrating, thinking, and remembering
____ Indecisiveness
____ Recurrent thoughts of death or suicide
____ Suicide attempts
____ Nervous exhaustion
____ Worrying excessively or being anxious
____ Frequent crying
____ Being extremely shy or sensitive
____ Lumps or swelling in your neck
____ Blurring of vision
____ Seeing double
____ Seeing colored halos around lights
____ Pains or itching around the eyes
____ Excess blinking or watering of the eyes
____ Loss of vision

___ Difficulty hearing
___ Earache
___ Running ear
___ Buzzing or other noises in the ears
___ Motion sickness
___ Teeth or gum problems
___ Sore or sensitive tongue
___ Change in sense of taste
___ Nose stuffed up
___ Runny nose
___ Sneezing spells
___ Frequent head colds
___ Bleeding from the nose
___ Sore throat even without a cold
___ Enlarged tonsils
___ Hoarse voice even without a cold
___ Difficulty or pain in swallowing
___ Wheezing or difficulty breathing
___ Coughing spells
___ Coughing up a lot of phlegm
___ Coughing up blood
___ Chest colds more than once a month
___ High blood pressure
___ Low blood pressure
___ Heart trouble
___ Thumping or racing heart
___ Pain or tightness in the chest
___ Shortness of breath
___ Heartburn
___ Feeling bloated
___ Excess belching
___ Discomfort in the pit of your stomach
___ Nausea
___ Vomiting blood
___ Peptic ulcer
___ Change in appetite
___ Digestive problems

___ Excessive hunger
___ Getting up frequently at night to urinate
___ Urinating more than 5–6 times a day
___ Unable to control your urine
___ Burning or pains when you urinate
___ Black, brown, or bloody urine
___ Difficulty starting your urine
___ Constant urge to urinate
___ Constipation
___ Diarrhea
___ Black or bloody bowel movement
___ Grey bowel movement
___ Pain when you move your bowels
___ Bleeding from your rectum
___ Stomach pains which double you up
___ Frequent stomach trouble
___ Intestinal worms
___ Hemorrhoids
___ Yellow jaundice
___ Biting your nails
___ Stuttering or stammering
___ Any kind of problem with your genital or sexual organs
___ Sexual problems
___ Hernia or rupture
___ Kidney or bladder disease
___ Stiff or painful muscles or joints
___ Swelling joints
___ Pain in your back or shoulders
___ Painful feet
___ Swelling in your armpits or groin
___ Trouble with swollen feet or ankles
___ Cramps in your legs at night or with walking
___ Itching or burning skin
___ Rash or pimples
___ Excess bleeding from a small cut
___ Easy burning skin
___ Dizziness or light headedness

___ Feeling faint or fainting
___ Numbness in any part of your body
___ Cold hands or feet even in hot weather
___ Paralysis
___ Blacking out
___ Fits, convulsions, or epilepsy
___ Change in your handwriting
___ Tendency to shake or tremble
___ Tendency to be too hot or too cold
___ Sweating more than usual
___ Hot flashes
___ Being short of breath with minimal effort
___ Failure to get adequate exercise
___ Being overweight
___ Being underweight
___ Having lost more than half of your teeth
___ Bleeding gums
___ Badly coated tongue
___ A lot of small accidents or injuries
___ Varicose veins
___ Headaches
___ Other aches and pains
___ Feeling pessimistic or hopeless
___ Have had any kind of surgery within the past year
___ Being upset easily by criticism
___ Having little annoyances get on your nerves and make you angry
___ Getting angry easily
___ Getting nervous around strangers
___ Feeling lonely
___ Having difficulty relaxing
___ Being troubled by frightening dreams or thoughts
___ Being disturbed by work or family problems
___ Wishing that you could get psychological or psychiatric help
___ Being tense or jittery
___ Being easily upset
___ Being in low spirits
___ Being in very low spirits

___ Believing that your life is out of your hands and controlled by external forces

___ Feeling that life is empty, filled with despair

___ Having no goals or aims at all

___ Having failed to make progress towards your life goals

___ Feeling that you are completely bound by factors outside yourself

___ Feeling sad, blue, or down in the dumps

___ Feeling slowed down or restless and unable to sit still

___ Frequent illness

___ Being confined to bed by illness

For men only:

___ Having a urine stream that's very weak or very slow

___ Having prostate trouble

___ Having unusual burning or discharge from your penis

___ Having swelling or lumps in your testicles

___ Having your testicles painful

___ Having trouble getting erections (getting hard)

For women only:

___ Having trouble with your menstrual period

___ Bleeding between your periods

___ Having heavy bleeding with your periods

___ Getting bloated or irritable before your periods

___ Taking birth control pills (in the last year)

___ Having lumps in your breasts

___ Having excess discharge from your vagina

___ Feeling weak or sick with your periods

___ Having to lie down when your periods start

___ Feeling tense and jumpy with your periods

___ Having constant hot flashes and sweats

___ Have had a hysterectomy or on hormonal replacement

TOTAL SYMPTOMS _____

If you have more than ten symptoms, the time has come to make some intelligent decisions about your lifestyle! And if you have over twenty symptoms, you may well already have significant maladaptation or illnesses!

Even without significant symptoms, it is wise to consider by age 30 some tests that might help you avoid major illnesses later:
- Complete blood count—red blood cells, white blood cells, platelets, etc.
- Chem panel—electrolytes, cholesterol, liver, and kidney functions, etc.
- Homocysteine—this should be 7.5 or LESS. Anything higher increases risk of heart attack, stroke, and cancer.
- Cardiac calcium index—the simplest, safest, least expensive way to be sure you are not beginning the process of coronary arteriosclerosis

Susan Kobasa has been a major contributor to our understanding of hardiness—our resilience or tolerance of life stressors. Since so many people are not optimally healthy and suffer the ravages of stress, it is important to look at the foundation of a healthy life. Clinically, about 40% of Americans are depressed and a similar number are not truly happy—they have what I call a subclinical depressive miasma. In addition to the genes we receive from our parents, there is a social environment that is critical for health. Obviously, there are essentials such as air, water, food, clothing, and shelter. Without those, nothing else is even worth considering. The next most essential is nurturing, which should begin with conception. Therein begins the problem for the 40% of individuals who are conceived out of wedlock. Children of unwed mothers are much more likely to be born prematurely, have lower birth weight, and have many times more emotional and physical problems than children born to committed parents. In the 70s, Ann Landers wrote a column in which she reported that of the 10,000 individuals who had written her, 70% said that they wished they had never had children! This led my wife and me to write *To Parent or Not?* This implies that a huge percentage of parents are too stressed themselves to provide adequate nurturing to their offspring.

The minimum requirements for providing a child the essential nurturing:
- A committed relationship of both parents who want a child

- Optimal health habits while pregnant
- A healthy delivery without spinal or general anesthesia
- A nurturing home for **at least** the first seven years of life

Absence of any one of these situations leads to severe deficiency in oxytocin production, which is a problem in:

- ADHD
- Autism
- Anxiety
- Depression
- Addiction
- Borderline personality
- Inadequate personality
- Schizophrenia

There are of course many factors, but the outstanding finding in every one of these emotional/mental disorders is that oxytocin is deficient. And of course, major trauma at any age may block a previously healthy person's production of oxytocin, leading to PTSD, Post-Traumatic Stress Disorder. In fact, I consider virtually all depression and significant anxiety to be post stress! Interestingly, stimulation of the Ring of Air also raises oxytocin, the bonding hormone which is deficient in ADHD, Autism, Depression, Addiction, and even in Schizophrenia!

From a physical point of view, disorders/diseases fall into several diagnosable categories:

- Addiction
- Autoimmune
- Benign tumor
- Biochemical/metabolic
- Degenerative
- Electrical
- Endocrine
- Hematologic
- Hereditary/congenital
- Immunological
- Infectious—amoebic, bacterial, fungal, protozoan, viral
- Inflammatory
- Psychological: emotional, mental/spiritual
- Malignant tumor

- Parasitic
- Surgical
- Traumatic
- Vascular

Almost all of these have some inflammatory component and some biochemical abnormality as well as a variety of immunological disorders.

And these problems seem to be associated with significant physical locations related to the psychological/spiritual issues of the seven chakras of the body:

- **First**—All parts of the legs. Family issues
- **Second**—Low back (bottom of third lumbar spine through sacrum), abdomen from belly button down and pelvis. Sexuality, finances, and security
- **Third**—From the belly button up to the rib cage (1st through 3rd lumbar vertebrae); upper abdomen. Self-esteem and responsibility
- **Fourth**—Chest, heart, lungs, breasts; (1st through 12th thoracic vertebrae). Love and judgment
- **Fifth**—Mouth, neck, shoulders, arms and hands; (1st through 7th cervical vertebrae). Will power—ability to express needs and desires
- **Sixth**—Brain, eyes, ears, nose, mind. Reason and logic
- **Seventh**—Spirituality, soul, God

In other words, stress not only initiates a variety of biochemical abnormalities, but specific parts of the body and organs are also affected when the anxiety, anger, guilt, or depression are related to the specific issues of the chakras! The stress initiates inflammation in a specific organ which cascades into many biochemical dysfunctions and the wide variety of possible diseases. Now, the "physical" cause of disease does not in any way mean that there is not an underlying stress issue. In general, some current life stress elicits anger, guilt, anxiety, or depression, and it reminds you at a deep "unconscious" level of unfinished issues from a previous life! Then a cycle of lost memories feeds the underlying cauldron of worries and aggravates the situation.

Now that you have some understanding of the causes of all illnesses, the big questions are:

Are you ready and willing to examine the problems in your life and to make whatever changes are necessary to correct all health issues??

Are you willing to develop the absolute *essential* practices for optimal health?

- No smoking
- Maintaining a body mass index between 18 to 24
- Eating a minimum of five servings fruits and vegetables daily
- Exercising a minimum of thirty minutes at least five days a week

*Only **three percent** of Americans have all **four** of these practices.*

Having talked to thousands of individuals at my workshops over the past forty years who have come to hear about health, at most 25% of each audience maintains these four practices! All the drugs and surgeries in the world cannot substitute for common sense! As far as I can tell, health is far more important than any other aspect of life!

In addition to these four essentials, good sleep—a minimum of seven hours daily and for most people eight hours—is critical. In all of history, societal stress has been present— from natural stressors such as weather to political ones. Stress is inevitable. Thus, finding ways to cope with external stress becomes equally critical. Stress can be:

- physical—heat, cold, pressure, physical injuries, etc.
- mental/emotional—worry, anger, anxiety, guilt, depression
- chemical—toxins such as arsenic, cadmium, aluminum, lead as well as some 550,000 chemical pollutants released into the air, water, and earth every year and now 80% of all food sold in the U.S. is junk!
- nuclear—radioactivity has increased many thousands of times in the past seventy years

Physical stress is perhaps most easily understood, with heat and cold being obvious. And perhaps the most common serious physical stress injuries are created by a modern luxury—automobiles. Not that earlier travel by horse or on foot was without potential physical stress.

Mental emotional stress requires both proactive and corrective approaches. For instance, it has been shown that twenty minutes of deep relaxation twice a day reduces insulin requirement and adrenalin production by 50% for the entire twenty-four hours. (See *The Relaxation Response* by Herb Benson.) In 1929, Edmund Jacobson demonstrated that thirty minutes of *progressive relaxation* not only reduced stress but also actually improved 89% of most stress illnesses! And beginning in 1912,

Johanne Schultz demonstrated that *autogenic training*, twenty minutes daily, reduced stress illnesses by 80%. By 1969, the first of six volumes on *autogenic training* was published, with 2600 scientific references. Although I have examined the wide variety of mental approaches to stress reduction for over forty years (See my *90 Days to Self-Health*), *autogenic training* is still my favorite because of the tremendous research showing that athletes, students, business people, and those with most stress illnesses are managed well by this simple tool—coordinating the words with your slow breathing and creating visual images to reinforce the statements. Essentially, you get into a relaxed physical body position and repeat for about three minutes each of the following statements:

- My arms and legs are heavy and warm.
- My heartbeat is calm and regular.
- My breathing is free and easy.
- My abdomen is warm.
- My forehead is cool.
- My mind is quiet and still.

Get the sensory feedback, awareness from each part of your body—face, jaws, neck, shoulders, arms and hands, chest, breasts, abdomen, back, buttocks, pelvis, legs before and after twenty minutes of practice. Basically you can feel good and OK with no tense pain or discomfort and *no feeling* from each and every body part. The goal is the relaxed and OK feedback from each part! If after twenty minutes there are still areas that are not relaxed and OK, you can:

- Talk to the body part—e.g., My back is relaxed and comfortable.
- Love it—appreciate that part of your body.
- Tense and release the muscles in that part of your body.
- Breathe in and collect tension or discomfort from that part of your body and breathe out, releasing the undesired sensation.
- Breathe through the skin over that part of your body
- Circulate the electrical energy from your heels up the back to the top of your head as you breathe in, and circulate the electrical energy down the front of your body as you breathe out.
- Expand the electromagnetic field around your feet and gradually up around every part of your body, toes to head, seeing and feeling yourself in a capsule of living EMF (electromotive force) energy. Start with one sinch and expand gradually to 12 inches.

Three months of daily practice will retrain your brain and auto-nomic, automatic, nervous system. Then you may be able to continue with only five minutes daily.

Other tools for total body relaxation and balancing are:
- Good music
- Flashing lights at 1 to 7 cycles per second, such as the Shealy RelaxMate II
- Vibratory music, through speakers placed in the mattress
- Using chakra glasses—there are the 7 major colors—red, orange, yellow, green, blue, indigo, purple. Different strokes for different people—some people achieve much greater peace, using one they particularly like
- Hot tubs, saunas, or a soak in a regular bathtub, perhaps adding a few drops of lavender oil to the water
- Dancing or jogging
- Just walking or lying in nature
- Sitting in a copper pyramid or in front of a copper panel on the wall
- Developing and using a mantra: I am relaxed and comfortable, etc.
- Lying on a true magnetic mattress—MagneticoSleep is excellent.

Managing Chemical Stress

If you remember your total life stress, you can review the obvious chemical stressors in your life. Some come from common food/drink intakes like sugar, coffee, and alcohol. Others from your habits or those around you, such as smoking. Others come from society—the addition of chlorine and fluoride to drinking water.

According to many sources, the average American eats one hun-dred-fifty pounds of sugar a year. That is three pounds or forty-eight ounces a week or almost seven ounces daily. That is forty-two tea-spoons of sugar daily! That is over eight stress points. About half is high fructose sugar added to many packaged foods. Each teaspoon deprives you of all the B vitamins, chromium, magnesium, and vanadium and helps burn out your adrenal glands. And of course this is *added* sugar, not that naturally found in fruits, etc.! No added sugar is needed or good. If you are consuming more than five teaspoons daily, your long-term health is at risk!!

Perhaps caffeine is the next most common chemical stressor. For most adults one cup of coffee daily is probably quite safe, but even without added sugar, one cup of coffee adds one stress point. The chemical stress of fluoride and chlorine is, like all stress, additive. To make it simple, *no* chlorine or fluoride is good or healthy, and if you just consume them daily, you have added three hundred-sixty-five stress points a year, or thirty a month! Remember that any stress above twenty points puts you at significant risk!

Table sugar is the first *artificial* food! The first food from which *all* vitamins, fiber, and minerals were removed! White rice was the second artificial food, removing the essential fiber and vitamins, leading especially to B 1 deficiency or beriberi. About 20% of all calories intake in the world comes from white rice, essentially a great stress food!

Wheat or the "staff of life" has been more prostituted than any other food. First and foremost, white flour is deficient in fiber, vitamins, and minerals. Further it is *bleached* with bromine, a neurologic toxin, and, most critically of all, it is now over 90% genetically modified, including the addition of Roundup®—a serious poison to the actual seed itself! I strongly advise eating *no* wheat.

With the chemicalization of most food also comes numerous artificial foods such as MSG, monosodium glutamate, a known brain toxin and *artificially* hydrogenated or trans-fats, which we cannot metabolize. Thus all margarines are far more toxically stressful than any natural fat. Then come the truly artificial, toxic, unreal junk sold as food: aspartame, saccharine, Splenda®, Olestra®, and artificial flavors, colors, tomato sauces, chocolate, etc. *All of these add chemical poisons and stress to your body!*

In addition, many modern fabrics, carpets, paints, insulation materials, detergents, etc. are chemical toxins, providing daily stress and even changing the endocrine glands—especially many estrogenic substances which have seriously altered the entire hormonal system. The addition of antibiotics to animal foods further increases the overall chemical stress load. Finally, cars and factories emit millions of tons of toxic chemicals daily. And that does not include the addition of cigarette smoking! After sixty years of national effort to get rid of tobacco, 22% of adults still smoke, poisoning themselves and those around them.

Average city life is significantly shorter than rural life even with the
marked chemical pollution of modern farming. Every state is different.
(See http://www.measureofamerica.org/maps/.) In general, because of
a variety of health habits, Asian Americans are healthier than Cauca-
sians, who are healthier than Latinos, African Americans, and Native
American Indians. In Connecticut, for instance, Asian Americans out-
live the average American by eleven years! Average Americans live
seventy-eight years, with an average life expectancy being decreased
by twenty-two years. *Those twenty-two years lost come from smoking, obesity,
crummy nutrition, and inadequate exercise.* Not only do average Americans
lose twenty-two years of life, at least 75% of all the illnesses that shorten
life and minimize health are *preventable!*

3

Nutrition

Water

As an adult you should drink half your body weight in pounds in ounces of good water. For 150 pounds of weight, that means 75 ounces of water! If you live in a city, I strongly recommend a good filter to remove chlorine and fluoride, at least from your drinking and cooking water. Ideally, you would remove it from your bathing water as well. Coffee and tea do *not* count as water, although any caffeine–free herbal tea will count as water intake. Fruit and vegetable juices also do not count as water, as they have many other substances that require the water content for metabolism.

Antioxidants

There are many natural antioxidants in nature, and if you eat at least 80% of your food as fresh fruits and vegetables, you will probably get enough. A list of important antioxidants follows:

Anthocyanins—these great red, orange, and blue colored fruits and vegetables—are tremendous and should be part of every diet.

Ascorbic acid—the essential in vitamin C—was discovered by the great scientist, Szent-Gyorgi, who took 10 grams daily. For adults, I recommend 2000 mg, best taken with 1000 mg of methyl sulfonyl sulfate, 60 mcg of molybdenum, and 3 to 6 mg of bet 1,3 glucan. This combination, found in my Youth Formula, helps restore DHEA. More about that later. For serious illnesses such as bad viral infections or cancer, I recommend up to 100 grams of vitamin C IV in a Myers cocktail. Of course, that requires a physician prescription and administration!

Vitamin A—the best known vitamin A comes from fish liver oil, most commonly cod liver. *However,* larger doses of vitamin A, even 10,000 units daily, can lead to severe brain swelling. You actually need *no* vitamin A, but you do need the family of carotenoids, the best known being beta carotene. This family includes beta carotene, astaxanthin, and lycopene. All are precursors to vitamin A and are safe at very high doses. I prefer 25,000 units of beta carotene and 4 to 10 mg of astaxanthin daily. Lycopene and lutein are other members of the family and are, interestingly, increased in availability by cooking the most common source—tomatoes.

CoQ10 (Ubiquinone)—one of the major immune supporters. I prefer a minimum of 100 mg daily.

Flavonoids—another fruit/vegetable family of antioxidants
Polyphenols—the final fruit/vegetable antioxidants

Essential Vitamins

Vitamin A—See above

The B Vitamins

B vitamins are essential for metabolism in general as well as production of energy and most importantly for brain and heart function. Despite the rather miniscule RDA's suggestion, in today's stressful environment, I think adults will be healthier if they take an average of 25 mg of the major ones.

B1, Thiamine—deficiency of B1 leads to beriberi, optic nerve damage, Korsakoff's syndrome, peripheral neuropathy, and heart failure. Up to 1000 mg daily is safe. Thiamine is absolutely required for metabolism of carbohydrates and alcohol, excess of which lead to beriberi. Up to 400 mg daily is safe.

B2, Riboflavin—B2 deficiency leads to inflammation of skin, mouth, tongue, and lips and anemia.

B3, Niacin—B3 deficiency leads to pellagra, which was rather common in the early twentieth century, again because of excess carbohydrate intake. This deficiency has a broader neurological/mental harm than virtually any other B vitamin. However, even 100 mg may cause significant flushing and a burning feeling in the skin. Another form of niacin, nicotinaminde or niacinamide, is safe up to 1500 mg daily and may help arthritis symptoms and some schizophrenics.

B4—was once thought to be a vitamin, but it is "just" a critical component of DNA and RNA.

B5, Pantothenic acid—Pantothenic acid is primarily essential for energy, including proper metabolism of fat, carbohydrate, and protein In general, it is quite safe up to 25 mg daily.

B6, Pyridoxine is one of the most commonly deficient B vitamins, even those who take the so-called RDA. Carpal tunnel syndrome, menstrual problems, and coronary artery disease are all major diseases of B6 deficiency It is safe up to 100 mg daily.

B7, Biotin—B7 deficiency results from a really crummy diet and affects all aspects of mind and energy.

B8, Inositol is critical for function of brain, mind, and immune system. Up to 100 mg is safe.

B9, Folate (folic acid)—This is one of the most critical vitamins for function of mind, brain, and the integrity of the arteries. The RDA is ridiculously low, and it is safe up to 100 mg daily. Inadequate folic acid is a major contributor to homocysteinemia, a major cause of coronary disease, Alzheimer's disease, stroke, diabetes, and cancer, as well as malformations of babies. Blood levels above 7.5 are increasingly dangerous, and most labs ridiculously consider up to 14 "normal."

B10, PABA (Para amino benzoic acid)—B10 deficiency leads to many autoimmune diseases ranging from those affecting the skin, collagen system, and even the penis! It is safe up to 2000 mg twice a day and can help prevent sunburn.

B11, Salicylic acid—In general B 11 can be manufactured by the body if you have adequate intake of phenylalanine, an essential amino acid. It is essential for the entire DNA system.

B12, Cobalamine (also Methylcobalamine)—B12 deficiency is best known as the cause of pernicious anemia, which leads not only to anemia but also to damage to the spinal cord and brain. It is found *only* in animal protein! Vegans will inevitably develop B12 deficiency unless they take it as a supplement, and I like to remind them that it is still made by an animal—at the very least by yeast! Up to 5000 micrograms daily is quite safe.

Vitamin C (ascorbic acid)—Vitamin C is as critical as Vitamin D in supporting immune health. The RDA of 60 mg is insanely low, and I believe adults with less than 1000 mg daily are at great risk.

Vitamin D3—80% of Americans are deficient in D3, largely because of the ridiculous advice of dermatologists to avoid sun and to use sun blocker. If you take no other advice from this book, take at least 5000 units of D 3 daily if you are an adult over 135 pounds. Children should take at least 50,000 units once a month after age 2.

Vitamin E, (Tocopherols and, more importantly, Tocotrienols)— One of the most basic antioxidant vitamins, working synergistically with A and C. 100 mg daily of gamma/delta Tocotrienols are essential for virtually every essential body function.

Carbohydrates

Carbohydrates are the broad field of sugars and starches. Essentially we do not need *any* carbs as we can make them out of fats or proteins. Naturally occurring carbohydrates, in general, are good, but "refined" and "enriched" carbohydrates are *junk food*! Table sugar, white flour, and fructose are plain *rubbish*, and they are major contributors to diabetes, heart disease, depression, ADHD, and cancer.

Honey is a blend of natural glucose and fructose and is much superior to sugar, since it is sweeter and contains some amino acids and vitamins. Used in moderation by all except diabetics, it is the only sweetener I recommend.

Fats

In general, naturally occurring fats in healthy meats, seeds, and nuts are good for you. Artificially hydrogenated or "hardened" fats are seriously dangerous, poisonous *junk*.

Omega-3—Omega-3s are alpha Linolenic acid (ALA), Eicosapentae-noic acid (EPA), and Docosahexaenoic acid (DHA). They are the *essential* fats. Deficiencies lead to inflammation and every known disease! Best sources are wild salmon and grass fed beef and poultry.

Omega 6—The only healthy sources are nut oils, evening prim-rose, and black currant oils. Other vegetable sources such as corn oil, sunflower oil, safflower oil, cottonseed, peanut, and soy oil are to be avoided!!

Omega-9—These monounsaturated fats are not essential but in general are healthy, with the very best being from virgin olive oil and avocados.

Essential Amino Acids

There are nine really essential amino acids and one "conditionally" essential.

Histidine is needed to make histamine, as well as to stabilize he-moglobin and inhibit carbon monoxide. Those with allergies may be deficient.

Branched Chain Amino Acids: *Isoleucine, Leucine, and Valine.* These three are essential for building muscle and protecting cartilage, the "glue" substance that ties everything together, and for making and keeping cartilage healthy. Deficiencies weaken the immune system and increase the risk of anxiety and depression.

Methionine is a sulfur-containing amino acid which can be widely used but with inadequate folic acid, B6, and B 12 can lead to homocys-teine, which is highly toxic.

Phenylalanine is essential for making the major stress essential triad: dopamine, norepinephrine, and epinephrine as well as for main-taining muscle.

Taurine is the most prevalent amino acid in the body BUT is defi-cient in 84% of depressed patients. It works synergistically with magnesium to stabilize cell membrane potential. It is especially helpful in depression, hypertension, epilepsy, insomnia and anxiety. Up to 6000 mg daily may be tried.

Threonine is essential for making collagen, bones, teeth and preventing neurological spasticity. A major cause of deficiency is leaky gut!

Tryptophan is perhaps the best known amino acid as it is used to make serotonin, the most stabilizing mood neurochemical. Of course, you cannot make serotonin without B6, B3, and lithium.

Conditionally Essential Amino Acids

Arginine is critical for maintaining muscle mass and for production of nitric oxide, a chemical essential to every cell function, including energy, immunity, and blood pressure. After age 0 arginine loses its significant contribution to nitric oxide (NO), because it is needed to maintain muscle mass.

Cysteine can usually be manufactured from methionine, if there are adequate amounts of B12, B6, and folate. It is a major contributor to energy.

Glutamine is made by healthy bacteria in the intestines and is also a "food" for growing more of the healthy probiotics which stabilize intestinal health.

Tyrosine is usually manufactured from the essential amino acid phenylalanine and would be deficient only in severe malnutrition.

Glycine is again a general malnutrition problem, as it is in all quality protein foods.

Ornithine deficiency is another general malnutrition problem. It works synergistically with arginine to assist in enhancing growth hormone release.

Proline is made in the body if there is not malnutrition. It is essential for maintaining cartilage.

Serine is manufactured from glycine and is deficient only in malnutrition.

There are a number of other amino acids which will be deficient only in general malnutrition—alanine, asparagine, aspartic acid, and glutamic acid.

Minerals

Calcium *is one of the mega minerals and in adults requires an intake of about 1000 mg daily.* However, if you take adequate vitamin D 3 and eat a good diet, you do not need supplements.

Carbon is a building block for all organic matter.

Chlorine is ordinarily eaten as salt and very few people will be deficient if they eat a wide variety of foods. Excess salt can cause hypertension and related diseases

Hydrogen is another building block of organic matter.

Magnesium is needed in over 350 enzymes and is second only to potassium and calcium in quantity. It is deficient in 80% of Americans because of high carbohydrate junk food and inadequate magnesium in the soil. It is far better absorbed through the skin than orally.

Phosphorus is prominent in all foods and would be deficient only in severe malnutrition. Soda pop, a major junk food, is loaded with excess phosphorus.

Potassium is the third of the major minerals and comes mostly from fruits and vegetables.

Sodium deficiency would ordinarily occur only in malnutrition. Excess occurs because of overabundance of salt in many packaged foods.

Sulfur comes mainly from the sulfur containing amino acids and as methyl sulfonyl sulfate. It is essential for supporting joints, cartilage, and making DHEA.

Trace Minerals

Boron is essential for preventing inflammation, for making testosterone, and for keeping bones strong. Most adults should take 9 mg.

Chromium is primarily necessary for production of insulin.

Cobalt is essential for making blood and balancing brain/mind.

Copper is mainly an anti-inflammatory and is a balancer with zinc.

Iodine is essential for this is deficient in 80% of Americans. It is essential for thyroid function, energy, and immune strength.

Iron is best known for its role in hemoglobin.

Lithium is critical for making serotonin and stabilizing mood.

Manganese is critical for brain function.

Molybdenum is needed for many enzyme functions.
Selenium is needed for immune strength.
Silicon is important for strong bones.
Vanadium is critical to prevent diabetes and hypertension.
Zinc is essential for immune strength and general overall metabolic balance.
Toxic Minerals *should be avoided!* These include aluminum, arsenic, cadmium, fluoride, lead, mercury, and uranium.

Artificial and Processed Additives

*The food industry has prostituted our food supply for the last century and created all these **junk** products:*
Artificial flavors, aspartame, high fructose corn syrup, margarine, monosodium glutamate, Olestra®, Splenda®, and "American" or processed cheese! *Avoid all!!*
The body is essentially alkaline—it has a pH that is above neutral. Blood and saliva should have a pH of 7.4. Urine, which gets rid of many waste products, should be acid at a pH 5.5 to a maximum of 6.5. Therefore, you should choose at least 80% of your foods from the alkaline producers!

Fruits

For anyone who is not overweight or diabetic, two to three servings of fruit daily are excellent. In general, a serving is 4 ounces of fruit or 6 ounces of juice. They are best raw, second best frozen, third best canned or dried.

Acai	Acerola	Apple, Baldwin
Apple, Crab	Apple, Delicious, Red	Apple Delicious, Yellow
Apple, Granny Smith	Apple, Grimes, Golden	Apple, Jonathan
Apple, McIntosh	Apple, Rome	Apple, Wealthy
Apple, Winesap	Apricot	Avocado
Baba Ghanoush	Banana	Banana Melon
Bitter Melon (Gourd)	Black Cherries	Black Elderberries, Raw

Black Mulberries, Raw   Black Raspberries, Raw   Blackberries, Raw
Blueberries, Raw   Blueberries, Wild, Raw   Breadnut, Dried
Buffaloberry   Camu Camu   Cantaloupe Melon
Carob   Chokeberries, Raw   Citron
Coconut, Raw   Coconut Milk   Cranberries, Raw
Cranberry Juice   Cranberry Juice,   Currents, Black, Raw
  Cocktail   Unsweetened
Currants, Red, Raw   Currants, White, Raw   Currants, Zante, Dried
Dates   Figs   Gooseberries
Grapefruit   Grapefruit Juice   Grapes, American Red
Grapes, Black   Guarana   Guava
Guava, Green Apple   Guava, Pineapple   Guava, Strawberry
Guava Nectar   Hawthorne Berries   Honeydew Melon
Huckleberries, Raw   Key Lime   Kiwi Fruit
Lemon   Lemon Grass   Lemon Juice
Lime   Lime Juice   Lingonberries, Raw
Lychee   Mandarin   Mango
Mango, Dried   Mango Nectar   Mangosteen, Dried
Mincemeat   Moringa Leaves   Muscadine Grapes
Muskmelon   Nectarine   Noni Fruit Juice
Olives, Green   Olives, Ripe   Orange, CA (Valencia)
Orange, Florida   Orange Juice   Orange Juice From
                                                     (Concentrate)
Orange, Naval   Papaya   Papaya Nectar,
                                                     Canned
Paw Paw Fruit (See: http://www.Pawpaw.Kysu.Edu/Pawpaw/Cooking.Htm–Top)
Peach   Peaches, Canned   Peach Nectar, Canned
Pear   Pear, Asian   Pear, Balsam
Pear, Dried   Pear, Prickly   Persian Lime
Persimmon, Japanese   Persimmon, Native   Pineapple
Plum   Plum, Java   Plum, Red
Plum, Wild   Pomegranate   Pomegranate Juice
Pumpkin   Pumpkin Seeds, Dried   Quince
Red Elderberries   Red Raspberries   Rhubarb
Rose Hips   Salmonberries   Strawberries
                           (Cloudberries)
Sweet Cherries   Tamarillo   Tangerine

Tart Cherries   Tart Cherry Juice Concentrate
Watermelon   Wolfberries

All fruits except cranberries, plums/prunes, and rhubarb are alkaline producing, which is highly desirable.

Vegetables
Veggie Veggies—all are alkaline producing!

Argula, Raw	Artichoke	Asparagus
Bamboo Shoots, Canned	Basil, Fresh	Beets, Cooked
Beet Greens, Cooked	Beet Greens, Raw	Bell Pepper (Green)
Bell Pepper (Red) Roasted	Bitter Leaf, Egusi Soup	Bok Choy
Broccoli	Broccoli Slaw Mix	Brussels Sprouts
Burdock Root	Cabbage, Many Varieties	Cabbage, Ethiopian
Cabbage Kraut	Celeriac, Raw	Celeriac
Celery	Celery Flakes, Dried	Celtuce
Chicory Greens	Chicory Roots	Chives
Chives, Garlic raw	Chrysanthemum, Garland	
Chrysanthemum, Garland Boiled Without Salt		
Coleslaw	Collards	Collards Kraut
Corn Salad	Cress	Cucumber
Cucumber, Pickles, Dilol	Dandelion Greens	Dill Weed, Dill Seed
Dulse	Edible-Podded Peas	Eggplant
Eggplant, Pickled	Eggplant Ratatouille	Endive
Fennel	Fennel Seed	Fiddlehead (Ostrich) Fern, Raw
Fiddlehead Fern	Garden Rocket	Garlic, Elephant
Garlic	Horseradish, Prepared	Jicama (Yambean), Raw
Jicama (Yambean)	Kale	Kohlrabi
Lambs Quarters	Leeks, Raw	Leeks
Lemon Grass	Lettuce, Numerous Varieties	Gourd

Malabar Spinach	Napa Chinese Cabbage	Nasturtium Flowers
New Zealand Spinach	Okra	Onions, Many Varieties
Parsley	Peas, Sprouted	Peppers, Sweet, Many Varieties
Peppers, Jalapeno	Purslane	Radicchio, Rape Leaves
Rutabagas	Mixed Green Salad	Shallots, Sorrel (Herb)
Spinach	Sprouts, Alfalfa	Sprouts, Mung Beans
Summer Squash, Yellow	Summer Squash, Green	Swiss Chard
Tomatoes, Scores of Varities	Wakame, Seaweed	Watercress
Water Spinach	Winter Melon	Zucchini, Summer Squash

Grains—acid producing

Bran Flakes	Chia Seeds	Granola
Millet	Muesli	Oats
Oats, Rolled	Quinoa	Whole Oat, Groats
Rice, Black	Rice, Brown,	Wild Rice Long–Grain

Legumes—acid producing except for string beans, snap beans, and snow peas

Alfalfa Seeds, Sprouted	Edible Podded Peas	Garbanzo Beans (Chickpeas)
Great Northern Beans	Green Peas	Haricot Beans
Kidney Beans	Lentils	Navy Beans
Peanuts	Peanut Butter, Natural	Snap Beans
Snow Peas, Sugar Peas	String (Green) Beans	

Mushrooms

Cordyceps Mushrooms	Morel Mushroom	Oyster Mushrooms

Portobello Mushroom   Reishi Mushrooms   Shiitake Mushroom
White, Button Mushroom

Eggs—acid producing
Eggs, Chicken, Duck, Goose, or Turkey

Dairy—acid producing

Cheese—dozens of Varieties	Kefir	Milk
Milk, 2%	Milk, Skim	Almond Milk
Coconut Milk	Goat's Milk	Soy Milk
Yogurt, Plain	Yogurt, Greek	

Meats—acid producing

Pork, many cuts	Beef, many cuts	Lamb
Rabbit	Chicken	Duck
Turkey	Goose	

Seafood—acid producing

Abalone	Ahi Poke Spicy Tuna	Alligator
Anchovy	Bass, Freshwater	Bass, Sea, Blackfish, Bluefish
Bream, Sea	Butterfish, Carp	Catfish
Caviar	Cisco, Smoked	Clams
Cod Atlantic	Cod Pacific	Crab, Alaska King
Crab Cakes	Croaker, Atlantic	Crappie, Wild
Devilfish (Alaska, Whale)	Dolphinfish, Raw	Drum, Freshwater
Eel	Flounder	Frog Legs
Gefiltefish	Grouper, Cooked, Dry Heat	Haddock
Halibut, Atlantic & Pacific	Halibut, Alaska, Cooked w/Skin	Herring
Ling Fish	Lingcod	Lobster
Mackerel	Mahi Mahi	Milkfish
Monkfish	Mullet	Octopus
Oysters	Perch	Pike

Pollock	Pompano	Red Snapper
Roe	Roughy, Orange	Salmon, Atlantic, Farmed
Salmon, Many Varities	Sardine	Scallops, (Bay & Sea)
Shark	Tuna	

Starchy Vegetables—acid producing

Beet (Beetroot)	Beet (Beetroot), Raw	Beet (Beetroot), pickled
Carrot	Carrot, boiled no salt	Carrot, Raw
Carrot Juice, Canned	Cauliflower	Corn
Ginger Root	Jerusalem Artichoke	Parsnip
Pumpkin, boiled no salt	Radish	Rutabaga (Swede)
Salsify (Vegetable Oyster), Raw	Sweet Potato	Turnip
Winter Squash, Many Varieties		

Spices–neutral

Allspice	Black Pepper	Black Tea
Borage	Burdock	Caraway
Cardamom	Chamomile	Cinnamon
Cloves	Cohosh	Comfrey
Coriander	Cumin	Dill
Echinacea	Fenugreek	Ginger
Ginseng	Green tea	Marjoram
Mint	Nettle	Nutmeg
Oregano	Red peppers	Rue
Sage	Himalayan Salt (far better than other salt sources, as it contains 3% trace minerals)	
Sarsaparilla	Sassafras	Sorrel
St. John's Wort	Turmeric	Willow Tea

Now, *with hundreds of different foods and scores of variety in preparation, you have no excuse for not having a minimum of 5 servings daily of fruits and vegetables, plus some quality protein!*

The exciting variations in preparing this potpourri of excellent foods are virtually endless. In general, your major concerns should be excluding artificial foods discussed earlier and avoiding the seriously dangerous GMO foods. Ideally, it is best to obtain as much as possible from real farmers who use no poisonous chemical pesticides or herbicides.

However, there is another widely prevalent substance in food that is potentially a serious health threat—lectins. At least 30% of all natural foods contain lectins, with the highest concentrations being in whole grains, peanuts, kidney beans, and soybeans. Tomatoes, eggplant, peppers, and Irish potatoes are relatively high, and it appears that sensitivities to these nightshades is very much an individual reaction and not nearly as universal as the problems with wheat. In addition to gluten, the other widely produced lectins are prime contributors to autoimmune diseases, such as Hashimoto's thyroiditis, rheumatoid arthritis, multiple sclerosis, etc. If your intestines contain enough natural mucin, the lectins bind to it and may pass unnoticed. If you are low in mucin, lectins bind to the intestinal linings and create serious bowel problems. Lectins include:

- Grains (wheat, quinoa, oats, buckwheat, rye, barley, millet, corn, and possibly rice, although most of the lectins in rice are not in the part that gets eaten)
- Legumes (any kind of bean plus peanuts, which have a particularly bad lectin)
- Soy

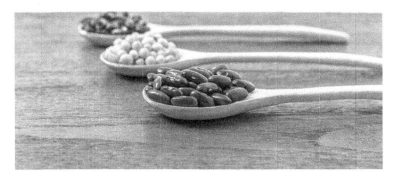

It's long been known that certain foods like kidney beans and castor beans contain especially toxic lectins. In fact, *the lectin Ricin, which is found in castor beans, is so toxic that it's used as a weapon in biochemical warfare.*

Current U.S. Department of Agriculture Vitamin and Mineral Recommendations

Micronutrient	Current DV[1]	My Recommendations
Vitamin A	5,000 IU	25,000 Beta Carotene
Vitamin C	60 mg	2000 mg
Calcium	1,000 mg	See Vitamin D
Iron	18 mg	18 mg
Vitamin D	400 IU	5000 IU
Vitamin E	30 IU	100 mg Tocotrienols
Vitamin K	80 mcg	100 mcg up to 15 mg
Thiamin	1.5 mg	25 mg
Riboflavin	1.7 mg	25 mg
Niacin	20 mg	25 mg
Vitamin B6	2 mg	25 mg
Folate	400 mcg	20 mg
Vitamin B12	6 mcg	1000 mcg
Biotin	300 mcg	300 mcg
Pantothenic acid	10 mg	25 mg
Phosphorus	1,000 mg	1000 mg
Iodine	150 mcg	1000 mcg
Magnesium	400 mg	Lotion
Zinc	15 mg	20 mg

Current U.S. Department of Agriculture
Vitamin and Mineral Recommendations

Micronutrient	Current DV[1]	My Recommendations
Selenium	100 mcg	10
Copper	2 mg	4 to 5 mg
Manganese	2 mg	2 mg
Chromium	120 mcg	1000 mcg
Molybdenum	75 mcg	75 mcg
Chloride	3,400 mg	3400 mg

The most critical advice of all in relation to nutrition is that 80% of your food should come from the alkaline fruits and vegetables and only 20% from the acid producing foods. Get yourself some pH paper, available at pharmacies and some health food stores. At least once a month check your saliva and urine pH to monitor this basic health state!

4

Exercise and Body Therapies

The physical body is designed to move. We are born with 270 bones, several of which fuse during childhood to become 260 in adulthood. When movement is inadequate, many bones become increasingly less mobile, stiff, and uncomfortable. We have 700 different muscles with their respective tendons, and muscle mass makes up about half of body weight in a healthy body. These essential energetic functions need not only movement but also resistance to maintain optimal health and benefit. A healthy body contains 12 to 15% fat. All nonextreme movement is good, and in our modern relatively inactive life, we need to provide a *minimum* of thirty minutes of moderate exercise five days a week. This can consist of:

- Limbering, calisthenics
- Yoga
- Sports
- Jogging
- Biking

- Dancing
- Treadmill
- Tai Chi
- Qi Gong
- Just bouncing in place—see bounce with Dr. Shealy on You Tube.
Also see my personal exercise program at:
www.youtube.com/watch?v=WtMVJ6yJaBs.
- A treadmill
- Health Rider®
- Weight lifting
- Walking
- A minitrampoline
- Jogging in a pool or hot tub

Ideally heart rate will at least double for half or more of your exercise period. There are a variety of vibrating plates, which provide a gentle but extremely beneficial addition to one's program. I use the Power Vibe® at least five days a week. In addition, Exercise with Oxygen Therapy, breathing 95% oxygen while exercising, adds considerable benefit.

The *Over 29 Exercise Book* by Jeffrey Furst is an excellent program utilizing the movements recommended by Edgar Cayce.

The following are suggestions Mr. Cayce gave in readings about exercise:

Q. State in detail what kind and amount of exercise the body should take?
A. As much outdoor exercise as is possible, always, for the body. A sufficient amount of *mental* exercise to keep an even keel or balance with that of the physical body; for the body nominally is an *active* body, mentally and physically, and in the manner as will make the body *physically* tired; so may the body be made *mentally* tired. These are the even keel for *this* body, particularly: Walking, riding, any outdoor exercise *good* . . .   202-4

The best way to acquire the correct amount of pep is to take the exercise!   288-38

It's well that each body, everybody, take exercise to counter-
act the daily routine activity so as to produce rest . . .   416-3

. . . Standing erect, raise the hand[s] high above the head as possible, rising on the toes, then slowly bending forward until the
hands will almost or quite touch the floor. Do this slowly, but
do it at least three, four, five, six times, *very* slowly, stretching
upward and forward and downward.   555-8

. . . No better exercises may be taken than . . . the cat-stretch-
ing exercises, which includes, of course, being able—(put very
coarsely)—to do the split, be able to put the head on the feet, to
put the feet behind the head, to make the head and neck exercises
and all of those activities that may be said to be of the feline or
cat exercise. To be sure, in the present period, present development, present conditions that exist, must be gone at gently; but
be persistent morning and evening, working at it, still not letting
it become rote, but purposeful.   681-2

Of morning, and upon arising especially (and don't sleep too
late!)—and before dressing so that the clothing is loose or the
fewer the better—stand erect before an open window, breathe
deeply, gradually raising hands *above* the head, and then with
the circular motion of the body from the hips bend forward;
breathing *in* (and through the nostrils) as the body rises on
its toes—breathing very deep; *exhaling suddenly* through the
mouth, not through the nasal passages. Take these {*exercises*} for
five to six minutes. Then as these progress, gradually *close* one
of the nostrils (even if it's necessary to use the hand—but if it is
closed with the left hand, raise the right hand; and when closing
the right nostril with the right hand, then raise the left hand) *as*
the breathing *in* is accomplished . . .
    . . . Then of an evening, just before retiring—{*with the body
prone, facing the floor and*} with the feet braced against the wall,
circle the torso by resting on the hands. Raise and lower the
body not merely by the hands but more from the torso, and with
more of a circular motion of the pelvic organs to strengthen the

muscular forces of the abdomen. Not such an activity as to cause
strain, but a gentle circular motion to the right two or three times,
and then to the left . . .   1523-2

. . . Exercise in the open air—as walking, as just sitting in same—is
necessary. Walking and swimming are the best exercises.
                                                             2164-1

. . . When ready to retire, let the exercise preferably be for the
lower limbs; this a movement as of sitting on the floor and
walking across, or swinging the limbs one in front of the other for three to four movements. Then in the morning, before
dressing, exercise the upper portion of the body; the arms up and
down — straight up, straight down; then the turning motion as
of swinging the arms around for the movement to the body from
the diaphragm upward . . .
{*When doing the*} exercises indicated; {*the focus*} of evening {*is*}
from the 9th dorsal downward; of morning from the 9th dorsal
upward. These will take away the heaviness and the tendency to
get tired easily.   2454-2

. . . Take this regularly, not taking it sometimes and leaving off
sometimes, but each morning and each evening take this exercise
regularly for six months and we will see a great deal of difference:
sitting erect, bend the head forward three times, to the back three
times, to the right side three times, to the left side three times, and
then circle the head each way three times. Don't hurry through
with it but take the time to do it. You will get results.   3549-1

Then, to give the body normal forces, and to bring the normal
effect in body, little of medicinal properties would be effective.
Better that climatic conditions; pure water {*carrying lithia*}, high
altitude. These, with food values, exercise of the physical body,
that the forces may be brought to exertion in the system, that the
body may become physically tired, without strain to the system.
Taking at such times exercises as would be given to the body
by deep manipulations to awaken the excretory system and the

secretive system through the liver proper.   3762-1

Morning and Evening Cayce Exercise Routines

The following is an in-depth explanation of the suggested Cayce exercise routines taken from
www.choosing-natural-health.com/cayce-exercises.html.

Morning Cayce Exercises
This set assists the day/night cycle our bodies require. That's why the morning ones are done standing, after lying down all night. They help us snap on to the day.

(1) **Bend and swing**—*An upper-body exercise that improves circulation, renews the air in the lungs, and adjusts the spinal column.*
   • Stand with feet flat on the floor.
   • Bend forward and swing the arms and upper body down and back up, with a rocking motion. Your fingertips should almost brush your toes on the downswing. Be careful of your balance until you're used to it.
   • Exhale on the downswing, inhale on the upswing.
   • Some people combine this exercise with (2) "Reach for the Sky" (below), going straight up into it on the upswing.

(2) **Reach for the Sky**—*Improves circulation and arches, naturally adjusts the spinal column, and is famous as an outer hemorrhoids cure.*
   • In a standing position (without shoes) gradually rise up on the balls of the feet, raising your arms in front of you at the same time, until they are as high as you can reach. Again, breathe in as you go up.
   • Still stretched out, slowly bend forward from the waist, with a clutching-the-air motion as you come down, until you can touch the floor. Breathe out as you go down.
   • Repeat this at least 3-4 times at first, and work up to 10-12.

(3) **Swing arms**—*Improves circulation to arm, and keeps joints limber and uncalcified—good for arthritis.*

- Stand with your feet apart.
- Swing each arm slowly in a circle, like a windmill—first one direction, then the other. Increase speed to your comfort level. I always imagine a pitcher winding up to throw.
- Keep your arms as relaxed as possible while you rotate them.
- I would begin with 10 times each way, unless you're already in shape.

(4) Rotate legs—*Good for the equilibrium and circulation, and keeps the joints limber.*
- Stand with spine straight.
- Lift one leg at a time, and rotate with the toes pointing outward. See yourself drawing a circle with your toes.
- Rotate each direction. Steady yourself by holding on to something, if you need to. Once you're used to it, try to balance yourself.
- At first, do 5–10 each way, and work up to your comfort level.
- Dr. Harold Reilly also suggests a variation with toes pointing up and heel down, while rotating. I do both.

(5) Neck Rolls—*Improves eyesight, hearing, circulation to the brain, and helps relieve stress. Cayce even said it would assist the thyroid.*
- In the morning, stand with feet spread slightly, and hands on hips.
- Keeping the spine straight, bend the neck slowly—forward three times, back three times, left three times, right three times.
- Next, roll the neck gently in a full circle, first one direction, then the other. Do this two or three times.
- For all you stiff necks out there, who have lots of tension, be careful! You can pull some muscles by going too fast or forcing. Relax . . . And if it hurts, don't push it—slow down even more and try to slide past it. (The rubberneck!)
- The safest way I've found is to make the neck muscles follow the eyes. This is very natural, since the neck is designed to turn wherever the eyes look.

Evening Cayce Exercises
Watch videos of all the Cayce Exercises!
The evening exercises are done in a basically horizontal position, after being upright all day. It signals the body to relax for the night. Cayce gave them for insomnia, among other things.

(6) Sitting sit-ups—*Improves circulation and stretch legs.*
- Sit on the floor.
- Touch toes repeatedly, rocking back and forth.
- Do 5-10.

(7) Cat walk—*Clears up the sinuses, improves circulation and general mobility. Keeps you spry!*
- Get down on all four paws.
- Imagine that you are a cat, and try to walk fluidly like one. This takes some practice.
- In addition to the daily routine, I do this whenever I'm congested, for quick relief. Cayce said this position was effective because early primates walked on all-fours—and didn't suffer from colds.

(8) Torso-circles—*Keeps the colon healthy, using centrifugal force to improve circulation in the colon, and strengthen its walls. This Cayce exercise is famous as an inner hemorrhoids cure, but is also very good for general health and longevity.*
- Put your body in a push-up position, with the soles of your feet against a wall or other solid object.
- Rotate your torso, first one direction, and then the other. Do equal numbers of these.
- I find it helps to hold your stomach in (if you can) while pushing with your feet on the wall.
- Don't do very many at first, especially if you're out of shape or overweight—even two or three in each direction are adequate to begin with. You can gradually increase 5-10-20 each way (or more for severe cases of piles).

(9) Bear walk—*Helps reverse the daily effects of gravity, improves circulation to the head, and loosens hip joints, in particular.*

- Stand with feet flat on the floor.
- Lean forward and put palms flat on the floor as well. Try to keep the feet as flat as possible, with legs straight, not bent at the knees.
- Holding this position, walk forward and backward across the room. This will be difficult, at first, since many people have trouble touching their toes. But after daily efforts, you'll be able to amble around like a bear.

(10) Neck Rolls—*These are the same as in (5) above, except that in afternoon or evening, Cayce recommended a sitting position, either on the ground, legs crossed (lotus, half lotus, or casual), or sitting on a bench or chair.*

There are numerous types of massage, the best being that developed by Dr. Harold Reilly amplifies the benefits of the Cayce exercises are listed here. There is a huge volume of information and recommendations to specific people for particular problems. (See Dr. Harold J. Reilly's book, *Handbook for Health through Drugless Therapy*, for more, or connect with the *A.R.E. database online*.)

Cayce also recommended massage and said that an hour of massage is worth four hours of sleep! There are numerous massage techniques, and some of the best are those developed by Dr. Harold Reilly. Personally, I think a massage a week is ideal, especially for those over fifty years of age. In addition, there are many other body therapies, including myofascial work, Rolfing, Schnelle work, Bowen Work, etc.

Hot soaks in a regular bathtub, especially with added magnesium chloride crystals, are also excellent for the body. Saunas and steam rooms as well as hot tubs all provide health benefits. My favorite detox approach is a castor oil bath, an elaboration of the castor oil pack often recommended by Cayce. Fill a bathtub with pleasantly hot water, splash into it one cup of castor oil and soak. Or you can rub castor oils over all your body neck to ankles and soak. To complete this safely, drain the tub and use a real shampoo to wash carefully the tub and your entire body *twice* before getting out of the tub. Alternatively, after a bath or shower dry off and rub your body from neck to ankles with castor oil and wear an old sweat suit all night. Local castor oil packs are particularly excellent for most abdominal problems and ankle, knee, or joint problems.

Although there is no substitute for physical exercise, massage is a wonderful adjunct, which I highly recommend. In addition, for some more stubborn muscle and joint problems, both chiropractic and osteopathic adjustments can be rejuvenating and sometimes virtually lifesaving. There is one problem that can be corrected *only* by one of the 10% of osteopaths who are real osteopaths. That is, 90% of DOs today do not do OMT, osteopathic manipulative therapy. I have seen hundreds of patients with a sacral shear, a rotation of the sacrum in two directions. I learned this diagnosis and treatment because in 1982 I developed a sacral shear and was blessed to have a young DO correct the problem. Virtually all the patients I have seen with a sacral shear have seen a chiropractor; and, unfortunately, chiropractors do not diagnose or treat this problem. Therefore, if you have low-back or buttocks pain and it is not corrected within a maximum of two or three chiropractic adjustments, find a DO who does OMT—do *not* bother seeing a DO who does not do OMT! And I am the only MD I know who checks for this problem. Of importance in this issue is the excess diagnosis of ruptured intervertebral disc. In 1972, I reviewed all the original records—history, x-rays, myelograms, and operative notes—on 250 patients referred to me for pain control after failed back surgery. I found that 80% of them had never had a real ruptured disc! Ten percent did have a ruptured disc, and in 10% I could not be certain with the available records. The point of this is that you should virtually never have back surgery just for back pain. Only when there is definite weakness or numbness should spinal surgery be considered. Personally, I believe that only experienced neurosurgeons should ever do disc surgery, not orthopedic physicians. And a fusion of the lumbar spine should be done only when there is a significant fracture or dislocation!

To a great extent, the same is true for cervical discs, except here an anterior interbody fusion may be the procedure of choice, depending on the judgment of the neurosurgeon.

The other common problem associated with the skeleton is degeneration of joints, especially the hip. Ideally, the best approach is to prevent such degeneration. This is best done by taking vitamin D 3, a minimum of 5,000 units daily in adults with at least 100 mcg of vitamin K 2, and using magnesium lotion, since our food supply is highly deficient.

Halitosis is better than no breath at all; any movement is better than no movement! If I still have not convinced you to move on your own, then consider a Chi Machine, which at least gives some body movement passively or a Power Vibe®, one of many devices that move for you. All you have to do is stand or lie on them!

Body Therapies

Beyond essential physical exercise, there are many health enhancing physical body therapies which include:
- Massage—many varieties
- Myofascial work
- Rolfing
- Alexander Technique
- Polarity therapy
- Chiropractic adjustments
- Osteopathic manipulation and adjustments
- Hydrotherapy—hot tubs, steam rooms, etc.
- Saunas
- Reiki
- Acupressure
- Acupuncture

Passing a "Fitness Center" this came to mind—

Fitness Center=Centering on fitness and pondering what it means to be fit

and—also— *Fitness Sent Her (and with wisdom keeps her going in the right direction.)*

I do not respond well to the noise, the classes, the flailing of bodies, the spinning, the loud booming music often found at the "gym." So many seem unaware of what they are doing and if they are doing "it" right . . . ear budded pushers . . . pushing while distracting themselves perhaps or straining to do . . . what? I *still* recall an Asian gentleman (well before I studied holistic medicine, traditional Chinese medicine, spirit–mind–body medicine, etc.) who exercised at the gym in Iowa City over thirty years ago. He was poetry in motion and his beautiful "work out" was a result of what had (I imagined) **been worked first from within.** He continues to be an example that I want to follow unlike so much of what I observe today . . . period. I see so few like him, and I find that unsettling. But I can only do what I can do!

In addition, there are a wide variety of electrical therapies, including the violet ray, the impedance device, and the wet-cell battery. All of these can be helpful in restoring body function when exercise alone is not adequate.

5

Mood, Personality, Beliefs, Values, Attitudes, and Emotions

Mood

State of mental feeling at a given time.

Personality

The broad concept of an individual's personal, social, and interactive skills or lack thereof. There are scores of "tests" that help to define various components of personality, with one of the broadest being the IPIP, the International Personality Item Pool, with 230 subdivisions. I include these, not just to be comprehensive, but for your careful introspection. Don't just skip these—stop as you read each word and ask yourself "Does this fit me?" **In fact, I suggest you put a little checkmark by each which *feels* like you.**

For Introductory Information about IPIP NEO-PI and personal Psu, visit
www.personal.psu.edu/j5j/IPIP/.
For the items in each of the preliminary IPIP scales
measuring constructs similar to those in the NEO–PI-R, see
http://ipip.ori.org/newNEOKey.htm .

IPIP NEO–PI

Achievement–striving	Activity–level (Adaptability)	Adventurousness
Aesthetic	Appreciation/Artistic	Affective Lability
Agreeableness	Altruism	Amiability
Anger	Anhedonia	Anxiety
Assertiveness	Attention to Emotions	Attractiveness
Authenticity/Integrity/ Honesty	Belligerence	Bravery/Courage/ Valor
Callousness	Calmness	Capacity for Love
Cautiousness	Cheerfulness	Citizenship/ Teamwork
Cognitive Failures	Cognitive Problems	Compassion
Competence	Complexity	Comprehension
Conformity	Conscientiousness	Conservatism
Cool–headedness	Cooperation	Courage/Bravery Valor
Creativity/Originality	Culture	Curiosity
Deliberateness	Dependence	Depression
Diligence	Disorderliness	Dissociation
Distrust	Docility	Dutifulness
Efficiency	Emotional Detachment	Emotional/Social Personal Intelligence
Emotional Stability; Emotionality	Emotion–based Decision–making	Empathy
Enthusiasm/Zest/ Vitality	Equity/Fairness	Excitement–seeking
Exhibitionism	Expressiveness	Extravagance
Extraversion	Fairness/Equity	Fantasy Proneness
Fearfulness	Femininity	Flexibility

Forcefulness	Forgiveness/Mercy	Friendliness
Gentleness	Generosity/Kindness	Good Nature
Grandiosity	Gratitude	Greed Avoidance
Gregariousness	Happiness	Harm-avoidance
Health Anxiety	Honesty/Integrity/ Authenticity	Hope/Optimism
Hostile Aggression	Humility/Modesty	Humor/Playfulness
Imagination	Immoderation	Imperturbability
Impression- Management	Impulse-control	Independence
Industriousness/ Perseverance Persistence	Ingenuity	Initiative
Inquisitiveness	Insight	Integrity/Honesty Authenticity
Intellect	Intellectual Breadth	Intellectual Complexity
Intellectual Openness	Introspection	Introversion
Irrational Beliefs	Irresponsibility	Joyfulness
Judgment/Open- Mindedness	Kindness/Generosity	Leadership
Learning, Love of	Liberalism	Liveliness
Locus of Control	Love, Capacity for	Love of Learning
Machiavellianism	Manipulativeness	Mercy/Forgiveness
Methodicalness	Mistrust	Moderation
Modesty/Humility	Morality	Need for Cognition
Need for Order & Cleanliness	Negative Expressivity	Negative Valence
Neuroticism	Non-Perseverance	Non-Planfulness
Norm Violation	Nurturance	Obsessive- Compulsive Symptoms
Open-mindedness/ Judgment	Openness to Experience	Optimism/Hope
Orderliness	Organization	Originality/Creativity
Patience	Peculiarity	Perfectionism
Perseverance/	Personal/Social/	Perspective/Wisdom

Industriousness/ Persistence
Physical Attractiveness
Pleasantness
Positive Expressivity

Prudence

Quickness
Recklessness
Relationship Insecurity
Resourcefulness
Responsive Joy
Risk-taking
Rudeness
Self-acceptance

Self Harm

Self-discipline
Self-esteem
Sensitivity
Sociability
Social-discomfort

Spirituality/ Religiousness
Sympathy

Temperance
Tolerance
Tranquility
Understanding
Unusual Beliefs

Emotional Perseverance
Planfulness
Poise
Private Self-Consciousness
Public Self-consciousness
Rationality
Reclusiveness
Religiousness/ Spirituality
Responsibility
Rigidity
Romantic Disinterest
Satisfaction
Self-consciousness

Self-regulation/ Self-control
Self-disclosure
Self-monitoring
Sentimentality
Social Boldness
Social/Personal/ Emotional Intelligence
Stability

Talkativeness

Tenderness
Toughness
Trust
Unlikely Virtues
Unusual Experiences

Playfulness/Humor
Politeness
Provocativeness

Purposefulness

Rebelliousness
Reflection
Reserve

Responsive Distress
Risk-avoidance
Romanticism
Security
Self-control/ Self-regulation
Self-deception

Self-efficacy
Self-sufficiency
Sincerity
Social-confidence
Social Withdrawal

Submissiveness

Teamwork/ Citizenship

Timidity
Traditionalism
Unconventionality
Unpretentiousness
Valor/Bravery/ Courage

Variety-seeking	Vitality/Enthusiasm/ Zest	Vulnerability
Warmth	Wisdom/Perspective	Workaholism
Zest/Vitality/Enthusiasm		

Now you might want to make a separate list of all the traits that you feel are really you! It is very valuable to spend several meditation sessions reviewing and introspecting on these!! What are you missing? What might you want to change?

With this remarkable variety of personality traits, there are almost as many personality inventories. My personal two favorites are the **Myers Briggs Type Inventory** and the **NEO–Five Factor Inventory.**
The Myers Briggs is one of the best self-understanding of all tests: www.**myersbriggs**.org/...
You are either:
Extraverted or Introverted; Sensing or Intuitive; Thinking or Feeling; Judging or Perceiving I strongly encourage you to go online and test yourself!
The NEO (Neuroticism–Extraversion–Openness) Five Factor Inventory, https://www.123**test**.com/big-**five**-personality-theory/, is perhaps the most widely accepted and used personality test, with only five· major traits:
Neuroticism, Extraversion, Openness to Experience, Agreeableness, and Conscientiousness
Of these, *conscientiousness is by far the most critical for health and longevity.* The major aspects of conscientiousness are reliable, organized, thorough, responsible.

Beliefs

Opinions and convictions that a concept or statement is true! This includes ideology, dogma, creeds, credo, articles of faith, convictions, etc.

Values

The following **list of values** from www.StevePavlina.com is perhaps

more comprehensive than any other I have found. On his website he
gives permission to use his material without copyright restriction, and
I am most grateful for this lengthy list. Incidentally, he has a number
of other resources as well as a free e-newsletter.

Abundance	Acceptance	Accessibility
Accomplishment	Accountability	Accuracy
Achievement	Acknowledgement	Activeness
Adaptability	Adoration	Adroitness
Advancement	Adventure	Affection
Affluence	Aggressiveness	Agility
Alertness	Altruism	Amazement
Ambition	Amusement	Anticipation
Appreciation	Approachability	Approval
Art	Articulacy	Artistry
Assertiveness	Assurance	Attentiveness
Attractiveness	Audacity	Availability
Awareness	Awe	Balance
Beauty	Being the best	Belonging
Benevolence	Bliss	Boldness
Bravery	Brilliance	Buoyancy
Calmness	Camaraderie	Candor
Capability	Care	Carefulness
Celebrity	Certainty	Challenge
Change	Charity	Charm
Chastity	Cheerfulness	Clarity
Cleanliness	Clear-mindedness	Cleverness
Closeness	Comfort	Commitment
Community	Compassion	Competence
Competition	Completion	Composure
Concentration	Confidence	Conformity
Congruency	Connection	Consciousness
Conservation	Consistency	Contentment
Continuity	Contribution	Control
Conviction	Conviviality	Coolness
Cooperation	Cordiality	Correctness
Country	Courage	Courtesy

Craftiness
Cunning
Decisiveness
Delight
Desire
Devoutness
Diligence
Discipline
Diversity
Drive
Eagerness
Ecstasy
Efficiency
Empathy
Energy
Enthusiasm
Euphoria
Exhilaration
Experience
Expressiveness
Exuberance
Fame
Fashion
Fidelity

Firmness
Flow
Fortitude
Friendliness
Fun
Gentility
Gratitude
Guidance
Health
Heroism
Honor
Humility

Creativity
Curiosity
Decorum
Dependability
Determination
Dexterity
Direction
Discovery
Dominance
Duty
Ease
Education
Elation
Encouragement
Enjoyment
Environmentalism
Excellence
Expectancy
Expertise
Extravagance
Fairness
Family
Fearlessness
Fierceness

Fitness
Fluency
Frankness
Friendship
Gallantry
Giving
Gregariousness
Happiness
Heart
Holiness
Hopefulness
Humor

Credibility
Daring
Deference
Depth
Devotion
Dignity
Directness
Discretion
Dreaming
Dynamism
Economy
Effectiveness
Elegance
Endurance
Entertainment
Ethics
Excitement
Expediency
Exploration
Extroversion
Faith
Fascination
Ferocity
Financial
    independence
Flexibility
Focus
Freedom
Frugality
Generosity
Grace
Growth
Harmony
Helpfulness
Honesty
Hospitality
Hygiene

Imagination	Impact	Impartiality
Independence	Individuality	Industry
Influence	Ingenuity	Inquisitiveness
Insightfulness	Inspiration	Integrity
Intellect	Intelligence	Intensity
Intimacy	Intrepidness	Introspection
Introversion	Intuition	Intuitiveness
Inventiveness	Investing	Involvement
Joy	Judiciousness	Justice
Keenness	Kindness	Knowledge
Leadership	Learning	Liberation
Liberty	Lightness	Liveliness
Logic	Longevity	Love
Loyalty	Majesty	Making a difference
Marriage	Mastery	Maturity
Meaning	Meekness	Mellowness
Meticulousness	Mindfulness	Modesty
Motivation	Mysteriousness	Nature
Neatness	Nerve	Noncomformity
Obedience	Open-mindedness	Openness
Optimism	Order	Organization
Originality	Outdoors	Outlandishness
Outrageousness	Partnership	Patience
Passion	Peace	Perceptiveness
Perfection	Perkiness	Perseverance
Persistence	Persuasiveness	Philanthropy
Piety	Playfulness	Pleasantness
Pleasure	Poise	Polish
Popularity	Potency	Power
Practicality	Pragmatism	Precision
Preparedness	Presence	Pride
Privacy	Proactivity	Professionalism
Prosperity	Prudence	Punctuality
Purity	Rationality	Realism
Reason	Reasonableness	Recognition
Recreation	Refinement	Reflection
Relaxation	Reliability	Relief

Religiousness
Resolution
Respect
Restraint
Rigor
Sagacity
Satisfaction
Self-control
Self-respect
Serenity
Sexuality
Significance
Simplicity
Solidarity
Soundness
Spirituality
Stability
Stillness
Success
Surprise
Teaching
Thankfulness
Thrift
Traditionalism
Trust
Understanding
Unity
Valor
Vigor
Vitality
Warm-heartedness
Wealth
Winning
Wonder
Zeal

Reputation
Resolve
Responsibility
Reverence
Sacredness
Saintliness
Science
Selflessness
Sensitivity
Service
Sharing
Silence
Sincerity
Solitude
Speed
Spontaneity
Status
Strength
Support
Sympathy
Teamwork
Thoroughness
Tidiness
Tranquility
Trustworthiness
Unflappability
Usefulness
Variety
Virtue
Vivacity
Warmth
Willfulness
Wisdom
Worthiness

Resilience
Resourcefulness
Rest
Richness
Sacrifice
Sanguinity
Security
Self-reliance
Sensuality
Sexiness
Shrewdness
Silliness
Skillfulness
Sophistication
Spirit
Spunk
Stealth
Structure
Supremacy
Synergy
Temperance
Thoughtfulness
Timeliness
Transcendence
Truth
Uniqueness
Utility
Victory
Vision
Volunteering
Watchfulness
Willingness
Wittiness
Youthfulness

Attitude

The result of your beliefs and values is a disposition to respond positively or negatively. A predisposition or a tendency to respond positively or negatively towards:

- Suggestions
- Ideas
- Objects or things
- Persons
- Situation
- Life in general

Attitudes determine our emotions, beliefs, and reactions. Here you might pause to think about both positive and negative attitudes and how they affect your mood.

You might want to list both your positive and negative attitudes towards:

- Religion
- Politics
- Race
- Education
- Government
- Climate
- Family
- Friends
- Teachers
- Work/career

Emotions

According to Wikipedia, Robert Plutchik's theory says that the eight basic emotions are:

- **Fear**→feeling afraid. Other words are *terror* (strong fear), *shock*, *phobia*.
- **Anger**→feeling angry. A stronger word is *rage*.
- **Sadness**→feeling sad. Other words are *sorrow*, *grief* (a stronger feeling, for example when someone has died) or *depression* (feeling sad for a long time). Some people think depression is a different emotion.

- **Joy**→feeling happy. Other words are *happiness, gladness.*
- **Disgust**→feeling something is wrong or dirty.
- **Trust**→a positive emotion; admiration is stronger; **acceptance** is weaker.
- **Anticipation**→in the sense of looking forward positively to something which is going to happen. **Expectation** is more neutral.
- **Surprise**→how one feels when something unexpected happens.

And it is interesting that this list does not include *love* or even *like.*

Remember, also, that I think the only problem is *fear,* and the reactions are anxiety, anger, guilt, or depression and their many synonyms!!

Edgar Cayce's health readings emphasized attitudes and emotions more than all other factors. I first became acquainted with them through Jeffrey Furst's wonderful book, *The Edgar Cayce Story of Attitudes and Emotions.* Then I acquired the three volume Cayce works on attitudes and emotions, one of the greatest treasure troves in this field. The following are my favorite selections from this trilogy. All item in bold print are my emphasis!

Attitudes and Emotions: General
Part I
78-4   M.23   12/18/30

In considering the conditions and circumstances that confront, and that influence the body at the present, many and varied may be the manners in which the entity may view same. Not only as how circumstances, conditions and surroundings affect the mental attitude of the body, but how the body is affected by same, as well as the outlook upon life the body gathers from the study of, contemplation of, self's position in its various phases, and *how* same is affected by self's attitude *and* outlook towards conditions.

In advising one as concerning the manner of activity, or action toward conditions under such circumstance, much might be said as to *just* advice—as to do or *don't* do this or that. The *conditions* as to be *met* are—What is the view or attitude to be assumed or taken as respecting *definite* conditions as exist in the life, as to outlook mentally, outlook physically, relationships to others, others' relationships to self. These should be the first considerations. Not only as duties, not only as privileges, but also as opportunities.

Do not get this position, however, as to ever be condemning self *or* another for that as exists in one's own life. If this be of self's own making, then know better than do the same thing again. If felt of another's making, then use same rather as a stepping-stone for *better* understanding and application of self . . .

Q. Please give me any advice regarding the maintaining a more perfect mental and physical balance.

A. In that as outlined may be that as an alignment of thought in a manner and direction as will give the proper attitude for the body, and the entity, in its activity. *Not* as a *servile* attitude; *not* as one in a position of embarrassment; neither as one that would laud or applaud self for anything accomplished *within* self—either physically or mentally; but rather in *humbleness* of heart, mind and body to be a channel for an ideal of *whatever* making self may choose; were it only to *that* ideal of self's relationship to an individual, to self, or to the Creative Forces—for they are *one*, and each are a pattern of the other.

Controlling Anger
165–2   M.50   10/10/27

In the urge through Mars' forces brings that at times of the temper that has been subdued in part through that of self's will to apply that of love and forbearance, rather than that as would appear in the urge to enact at that time.

One that brings much confidence to others through the acts as carried out by self in development towards that idea set for self.

One that gives much of self for the enlightenment of others through that of love for fellow man, and for the expressing of that urge felt in that—sweets draw many more flies than vinegar. This often felt in self as true, that to show one to be worthy one must be worthy in self.

One that finds much in common with those that ring true,

and little in common with those who would climb up some other way.

One that enjoys the joke, the pleasure as expressed in clean wholesome fun, yet little in common with that that belittles or besmirches any individual as individual, or as race or people.

One that will give much understanding to others through the application of those conditions that bring the better understanding of application toward the ideal in the individual life, for to the entity—as the good is manifest—the body, the entity, good. To that as is of show or of any favor that besmirches or belittles self for position, power, or such—*these* are little in the eyes of the entity.

Beware, though, of expressions in the temper, or in the power of the body physical or mental over the weak for the urge often comes to exercise such. Never turn same for self's own interest, for—as will be seen through experiences in the earth's plane—much may be lost through aggrandizement of selfish motives. Little of self is held in esteem above others, would there be humble and the contrite heart before the Creative Forces that give—to others that the understanding of relations between men as men, or man's relation to the Creative Forces—for in selfishness is the greatest plague, the greatest hindrance, the greatest barrier towards man's own development. Hence beware of association or the contact of self towards those who would give their own bodies and souls for position, power, fame, or monies.

361-4   M.15   8/10/34

From Mars we find a tendency for the body-mind at times to be easily aroused to anger. Anger is correct, provided it is *governed*. For it is as material things in the earth that are not governed. **There is *power* even in anger. He that is angry and sinneth not controls self. He that is angry and allows such to become the expression in the belittling of self, or the self indulgence of self in any direction, brings to self those things that partake of the spirit of that which is the produce or influence of anger itself.**

412-5   M.30   3/16/32

The entity would be considered by *some* as a leader. *True*, provided there is someone, or thing, or condition, that is the urge or the impulse for the entity to go forward. Hence the entity may be said to be passing through, in this experience, that of a crucial trial, or test, as to whether he is a big man, a developed and developing soul, or one that would again partake of those flesh pots in the satisfying of the callings of the flesh as to make that apparently strong become weakness in itself. *Know*, then, in *whom* thou hast believed, and that the ideal is set in things on high, rather than in that where moth and rust doth corrupt and where obligations may be turned into selfish desires.

Those influences in Mars make for many accentuations of the mental, as well as the ability—or broadness—of vision. Too oft has the entity experienced that the impelling force at times was that of *physical* determination, that would not allow self to be downed by the activities of others. Grit, or "get-up"—termed by many. This is an element that may be both constructive and destructive in the make-up of an individual. **Woe to him who may be *ruled* by wrath.** Woe to him who is also of such a nature as to allow the temper, or the elements that make for impulses, to be so overshadowed by that as is momentarily necessary for the activities of a life and not grounded in Truth, that arises from *spiritual* concepts.

497–1   F.46   1/23/34

From Mars we find those influences that have made and do make for experiences where there are the activities accredited to Mars; in wrath, in war, in allowing self and self's associations—not of the *entity* so much as in the capacities and abilities of others to be attracted in the environs of the entity, to be influences that have had to deal with the experiences of the entity in the present sojourn.

In this relationship to the entity much has been gained, for with the application of the mental forces, as maintained in the activities of the entity in self; while not always serene in self, *outwardly* the activities have been to control self. **Wrath is rather an excellent quality, but wrath uncontrolled is very bad and very detrimental, as the entity has found even in the present experience.**

518-2   F.25   8/13/35

Then again, in the appearances, do not look or seek for the phenomenon of the experience without the purpose, the aim. *Use* same as a criterion, as to what to do and what not to do. Not that it, the simple experience has made or set *anything* permanent! For there is the constant change evidenced before us; until the soul has been washed clean through that the soul in its body, in its temple, has *experienced* by the manner in which it has acted, has spoken, has thought, has desired in its relationships to its fellow man!

Not in selfishness, not in grudge, not in wrath; not in *any* of those things that make for the separation of the I AM from the Creative Forces, or Energy, or God. **But the simpleness, the gentleness, the humbleness, the faithfulness, the long-suffering,** *patience!* **These be the attributes and those things which the soul takes cognizance of in its walks and activities before men.** Not to be *seen* of men, but that the love may be manifested as the Father has shown through the Son and in the earth day by day. Thus He keeps the bounty, thus He keeps the conditions such that the individual soul may—if it will but meet or look within—find indeed *His* presence abiding ever.

793-2   F.53   8/27/36

Thus we find the entity prone to be in its arguments very conservative, very orthodox. Yet in its thoughts, in its deeds, in its associations, it is prone to those forces in the opposite. And yet a student, a seeker; yet a home builder. And still confused. Why?

Know thyself! And then ye may know the greater relationships that each emotion brings in thine experience. When anger hath beset thee, has thou stopped and considered what the fruit of rash words would bring? Hast thou not rather said, "Yes, but

I forgive but I cannot forget. Yes, I will not remember but don't remind me of what you did."

How hath it been given? If ye would be forgiven, ye must forgive. If ye would know love, ye must be lovely. If ye would have *Life. Give* it! What is Life? GOD! — in action with thy fellow man!

956-1   M.23   7/20/35

The influences from Mars, as we find, make for one who may *oft* show its anger, its resentment, in associations, in those things that lie very close to the inner man. Yet there has been through the sojourns in Venus and Jupiter, brought to the attention of the inner self that fact: He without a temper or without resentment or without care may manifest very little. **And he that does not control resentment, he that does not control anger, he that does not control that urge for the egotism in self, is indeed worse that he has none; for such may make for stumbling blocks and experiences that bring distraughtness and disturbances, not only of self as to the** *thoughts* **of self but to the fellow man.**

For, as has oft been said in the experiences in the earth, unless the high ideal is set, or unless the ideal of self is set in the spiritual attributes that partake of the Creative Forces or energies that may manifest in or through men in their material activity, little of value or of worth may come — and less of growth of the soul for its return to its former state with and in the creative energies that may manifest in the spiritual, the mental or the material world. Unless the activities are founded in spirit of the Creative Forces, they must eventually come to naught.

1003-2   M.25   3/6/37

Those influences from Mars are rather unusual; for these as combined with the Jupiterian as well as the Uranian make for extremes in the experiences; and anger or wrath, whether in the material activity of self or of others, makes for a very definite change in the emotions, the mental attitudes; and unless held in abeyance in self has much to do with material applications.

Hence those influences that make for the expressions in anger should be much as may have been said by some, **"When anger arises, at least count ten before you speak."** That will save not only self but many regrets and many associations that are for a greater and more satisfactory experience in this particular sojourn.

1797-1   M.39   1/21/39

Affection is in the innate forces a part of the entity. To lavish same upon others close to self is the nature, as also the desire to have same lavished upon self. This well to be applied in the material associations also. For the soft word turneth away wrath, while grievous words stir up anger.

Learn to pour oil upon troubled waters, as water upon fire; and feed not that of hate nor animosity, for these become influences that may destroy the good that is purposed and is turned into forces that become destructive in their materialization in the experience . . .

The emotions of self, as indicated, are easily aroused through affection; whether it is to be for the holding of grudges, animosities, or for the evening of same by turning to the still small voice as may speak from within. Not merely as something to hide behind, something to use as an excuse, or in the attempt to justify self.

1819-1   M.39   2/13/39

The attitudes have much to do with the general physical conditions. Let the attitudes be more of a constructive nature; more of patience, more of brotherly love, more of "give and take."

Do not hold resentment. Do not get so mad at times when things are a little wrong.

Remember that others have as much right to their opinions as self, but that there is a level from which all may work together for good. Smile always—and *live* the smile!

1819-2   M.39   3/16/3

Q. Please explain from the last reading the following: "Yet when there is the allowing of the body to become upset, or to become antagonistic, or to take very decided sides in this or that direction . . . " The entity and his wife do not feel that he is like this at all.
A. Then he should better analyze himself—for those antagonistic feelings and influences have been and are, as we have given, a portion of the disturbing influences within the bodily forces of the body.

Q. Please explain, "constant resistance kept as through the holding of resentments, the creating of activities in the finding of fault here and there." The entity and wife feel that this is not true of the body.
A. Then they err. For insofar as these influences work upon the activities of the mental forces and influences about the body, they deter from the abilities of the body to express the full creative forces and influences in its activities as it might.

Q. Please explain: "Do not get so mad at times when things are a little wrong." This the entity feels that he does not do; he feels that he is tolerant of others' opinions.
A. **Then just** *don't* **get mad! The very idea or expression that he is not, shows his intolerance!**

Q. The body is not troubled with poor elimination and a gas condition as indicated. Please explain.
A. These exist from the general conditions which exist, because of the lack of proper eliminations from the system through the fecal forces of the body-influence itself, as we find. **If there is the dislike, or the resentment—then don't use it.**

1857-2   F.39   3/28/40

We find from Mars that the entity has a very good temper; this isn't bad temper, but a *good* temper! **One without a temper is in very bad shape, but one who can't control his temper is in still worse shape!** The entity is one, then, who has learned to *hold* the temper, and yet not be entirely suppressed in doing so—or by the needs of such; rather being able to gain from same, through the very virtue of patience and long-suffering, which has been and is the experience of the entity through this particular sojourn.

1912-1 M.18 2/18/31

Q. How can they best understand each other, to make for a happily married life?
A. Understand *self*; and knowing that—as their lives are builded again together, as of old, in a compatibleness that will be found in each—knowing that there must *not* be losing of temper (for both are high tempered) at the same time.

2148-7 M.2 11/19/42

We find the urges astrologically from Mercury, Mars, Jupiter and Uranus are a portion of the entity's experience. Venus is both afflicted and having an urge in combination with Jupiter. Hence we will find these are some of the characteristics indicated, and that will develop as the body-mind develops.
One always above its years in observation, interest and activity.
   One that can get as mad as the most, and becomes very determined in self. These are necessary, yet if these are not controlled by the entity they may become hard to deal with. **And the ability to control must be instilled in the unfolding mind of the entity. These are indicated in mind and in Mars, and will also bring strength and virility, and a strong body after those periods of the unfoldment have come.**

2486-1 F.22 4/3/26

One that has been often in the earth's plane; hence has many influences and urges that are in exceeding strength of the physical being.
   One given to the highest ideals, and the attaining of same through *mental* equipment first. One that has little patience with the ones who neglect this phase of mental development, yet one

who has the kind word for one of every position or station in life, yet one that does not often pity one of low estate or degree, yet there is little of the caste nature within the individual's make-up, for the worthiness and the abilities of an individual count first and foremost in the mental forces of the entity.

One, then, slow to wrath, yet when mad—awful, awful, mad! One that can control self in this respect to a great degree, yet when reaches the breaking point gets all mad at once, and draws, as it were, within self until an equilibrium, or until self has reasoned the conditions out again—then goes on as if it had never happened.

In this respect, then, we find there are many contrariwise conditions, apparently, in the make-up of the entity.

One that love has little to do within the life in an expressive way and manner; rather love by reason and by aptitude than by sentiment, yet there is much of sentiment, much of affection, in the nature of the individual, and the personality of the entity often is combative with same. In the deeper sense, however, this we find is the basis of much of the ennobling influences in the life.

One that *should*, however, steer clear of firearms, electricity, and of explosives of every nature, especially when in temper, or when allowing self to become overexcited in any manner (though the entity does not find self afraid of *anything*, see?).

2520-1   F.38   6/23/41

This is the manner ye may meet that urge which at times prompts thee to seek revenge. That belongs only to Him and is not of thyself. For, this brings or breeds hate. **And hate is sin.**

Anger—Effects on the Body
23-3   F.26   3/21/37

Q. Any other advice for the body at this time?
A. Keep in that of constructive thought; because, to be sure, the thoughts of the body act upon the emotions as well as the assim-

ilating forces. **Poisons are accumulated or produced by anger or by resentment or animosity. Keep sweet!**

272-1   F.32   10/29/30

In the nervous system, or systems—Here we find, from the *physical* sense, the *greater* amount of distress—for, from there being stored in the mental forces of the body those of aggression, discontent, the holding of the disorders against individuals, has produced much as has been stored as of detrimental influences; **for *anger* in the system destroys that characterization of a perfect, or even a well-*balanced assimilation*, which makes for *physical* impoverishments, and with the constant brooding brings depressions that affect especially the sensory system; eyes, ears, nose, throat.**

281-54   Glad Helpers Group   5/28/41

Q. Anger causes poisons to be secreted from the glands. Joy has the opposite effect. The adrenal glands are principally involved, reacting through the solar plexus to all parts of the body.
A. The adrenals principally, but *all* of the glands are involved; as: A nursing mother would find that anger would affect the mammary glands. One nursing would find the digestive glands affected. The liver, the kidneys and *all* glands are affected; though it is correct that the reaction is *principally* through the adrenals.

2337-1   M.58   8/29/40

In Mars we find at times anger, or not just having what's wanted at the moment upsets the entity. Curb this. **Know that all comes to him who puts his trust in the all-powerful influence of love and harmony, the real poem of life, and then works like thunder for same!**

3510-1   M.36   12/16/43

While there is much yet to be desired, the desired results or the best results may not be obtained unless there can be created a greater desire on the part of the body itself for the corrections of the conditions; the anger, the hate, the conditions to gratify appetites that so break down that administration which has been or may be made.

4290-1   F.58   12/2/25

In the blood supply, this, we see, in the abnormal condition more by the action of temper in the body that by the physical conditions, for with the over-taxation and poisons as are brought in the blood stream through this physical action in the mental state, all of the functioning organs come under the stress of same. Then we have poor assimilation, poor digestion, and the greater troubles as we find, that has produced this, being that condition as is existent in the throat and in the portion of the body affected by these poisons as are absorbed from that condition existent in the tonsil and in the portion of the body that is affected by the ductless glands of the body.

Antagonism
969-1   M.69   8/6/35

Q. Will the attacks come to naught that have been made on me by the American Medical Association?
A. Depends upon the antagonistic attitude that the body assumes, or as to what the determinations are in the self. If ye would be antagonized, then be antagonistic! If ye would have peace, be peaceful! If ye would have friends, show yourself friendly! If ye would be *wise*, be patient and humble; and don't talk too much. Talk in the proper place, saying the proper things; not that to satisfy but that being sought by all—the longing to know of the peace that may be had by the soul of man, that under any other name becomes the *one* great thing in the experience of every liv-

ing soul; to find harmony and peace, and to be assured *by* those that *experience* the continuity of existence.

1152-2   F.61   11/20/36

Q. Regarding the situation which has arisen between the friend who went abroad with me and myself. Please explain this, and how I can meet it.

A. These conditions arise from former differences of opinion. And there has been gradually built an antagonism that may only be melted with loving indifference.

This, to be sure, at first may be called contradictory. For how *can* there be *loving* indifference?

How gave He, thy pattern?

When there arose those experiences when others were called to His presence and they said, "See, these in thy name heal the sick, cast out demons, yet they gather not with us. Rebuke them." But what was His answer? "Nay; nay, not so—for they that gather not with us scatter abroad the praises. Leave them, lest they turn again upon *you* and use that thou hast done to thine own confusion."

Then thy attitude should be:

Lord, they are Thine, as I am Thine. I am willing. I forgive. I present the problems to Thee. Use me, use them, in whatever *may be Thy will in the matter.*

This then puts thee in that position that there is no stumbling block, and that becomes then *loving* indifference. For ye have left it in the hands of the Creator, who alone can give life and withdraw it.

Anxiety
830-2   M.20   1/2/37

Rather then let that counsel be as given, in purpose, in sincerity. Insist that this be held as the ideal: *Sincerity* in every activity, in every relationship. And whatever may be undertaken, do with all thy might, with an eye single to service to a *living* God that may *not* in *any* manner be set aside.

For it is in Him that each soul lives, moves and has its being. And while a man may defy the laws of nature, defy even the laws of his Creator, he must pay and Pay and *pay*!

For His purposes will not be defeated among His children.

And each soul must give an *account* of the deeds, of the purposes done in the body!

1319-2   F.56   1/22/37

In considering the material surroundings, as has been indicated the great anxiety which has been experienced has had much to do with the physical reactions in the body.

But those tendencies in the mental self to judge others, to hold malice, to make for condemning of others for their seeming lack of anxiety or for their seeming lack of attention to that which self holds as an obligation, do not make for peaceful or harmonious experiences.

1349-1   M.25   3/16/37

Q. Why am I always so tired and logey?
A. Too much expended in the way and manner as indicated; over-anxious—and this uses up the energy without taking in sufficient of that to make for the proper recuperation.

1472-7   F.58   10/8/38

Q. Am I in any danger of losing my present position because of continued poor business on the . . . and can I do more than I am doing to improve these conditions?
A. This as we find *apparently* is a problem to be considered. But such should not make for anxiety. If the conditions in the minds of those who manage same justify the changes, or alterations, or eliminations entirely—it should not make for such anxieties to the body as to undermine the better health vibrations.

For as is understood—anxiety is like fear, and is as canker to any disturbed *nervous* condition of a body, if it takes hold.

But rather do that the hands and the mind *find* to do; knowing that what is best—and that will give the greater opportunity for the self to be of greater service—will be thy lot; if that is thy purpose and if thy life is lived in that manner.

Appreciation
257-215   M.46   1/12/40

Now as we find, there only needs to be those precautions which have been indicated for the body so often; that there be not an overtaxing in *any* manner.

Do not attempt to drive self so severely, either mentally, physically or materially; but take the precautions as to diet, as to meat and drink, and as to becoming overnervous, overexcited, or overanxious.

Then we will find the need for budgeting the time for those recreations that have been indicated. These should keep the body, the mind, in such a way and manner as to be more appreciative of all that which has been the privilege, the opportunity of the entity, to be in accord and in touch with those sources of help and aid, for its activity. These should be appreciated, and these are influences that will aid better in the attitudes of every nature.

1094-1   M.18   1/4/36

Q. What should be my attitude toward my mother and her efforts in my behalf?
A. Much as that which has been indicated; that there are duties, there are obligations, there are privileges. The duties are to self; the opportunities or privileges are to show the *appreciations* of the efforts in thine behalf. Then, as the mother love expresses to each individual the closest kinship of creative force to the human experience, it is not as a duty, not as an obligation, but as an opportunity for appreciation!

For the most despicable experience in any life may be, before the Throne of Grace, lack of appreciation!

1857-2   F39   3/28/40

Q. How can I shape my life so as to make the greatest possible
spiritual advancement in this incarnation?
A. Study those things that have been the shortcomings, and those
that have been and that have brought the greater blessings in the
experiences through the various sojourns in the earth. Then magnify those things in which there is greater stress, and greater faith,
and greater activity toward bringing material as well as mental
and spiritual development. They are—as has been set—ever the
same. For the law of the Lord *is* perfect, converting the soul. It
reneweth a righteous spirit within thee, day by day. Meditate oft,
then, in those things and in those experiences.

For, much of that which was the activity through those various
periods, by thy own intuitive force, may be made better known
to thee; and as to how and in what manner ye may conduct self,
not only in relationships to others but as to conditions which
arise in the experience of those ye meet day by day.

Remember to keep that appreciativeness, not only for what
He is, has been and ever will be in thy experience, but that ye
may *glorify* Him in thy speech, in thy activity, in thy associations
one with another.

Belittlement
2460-1   M.40   3/8/41

Do not attempt to be in business for self; for you mistrust self too
oft. Let thy left hand know not what thy right hand doeth, oft.

**Do not belittle or condemn self. *Know* you are right—then
go ahead.**

2727-1   M.56   4/13/42

Before this, then, the entity was in the land of the present nativity,
in what was then known as Fort Dearborn; during those periods
when it became necessary for the evacuation—when there were
indicated the greater abilities of the entity. Just as in everyday ex-

perience, it is not the quiet period that brings always the real value or real development or retarding of an individual experience, but that period when anxieties of a mental, material or spiritual nature arise. For, as has been indicated of old, there is daily set before each individual good and evil, life and death. And man chooses; he chooses through the gift of the will from the Creative Forces. Thus each choice, each decision, should ever be tempered with *spiritual* purposes, and these apply whether in the trade relations, the marital relations, friendships, just acquaintances, or in the so-called business dealings or with the public. For, *this* is creative. And that which is creative grows. **That which would take advantage of or belittle the hopes of any individual, under any circumstances, is belittling, degrading, retarding to that soul entity who uses same.**

2775-1   M.49   7/1/42

One that is prone to belittle its own abilities; and this is so seldom found in the experience of individuals. Yet there needs to be, as is latent and manifested, a desire for expression of self and self's undertakings, as well as self's knowledge.

While some of the material experiences are prone to bring about this tendency for self-effacement as to expressions, as well as for keeping self in the background of things or experiences that it would aid or foster, we find that those should not be so much expressed.

True, one must become selfless, but to have knowledge and withhold same from others is not always best. True, the entity tends to depart from the beaten path, as it cannot stand to be confined by ritual for ritual's sake—or because it is someone's idea.

It is necessary for proof, to the entity, of its every activity; yet as a student, and almost as an adept in the awakening or unfoldment of the abilities within, there needs to be the expression.

Blame
2281-1 F.32 6/16/40

For, each soul comes into an experience not merely by chance but that it, the soul, may have the opportunity to be an expression, a manifestation of that force called God, in materiality.

For He hath not willed that any soul should perish, but hath given with every temptation, with every trial, that strength, that peace, that harmony which if grasped hold of makes all trials and temptations to be stepping-stones to a greater awakening, a greater awareness to the beauties and joys that await those who love the Lord and His coming.

So, with this entity—though the burdens and the trials have at times become heavy, and though they may become heavy at the suddenness, the unusualness of the character or kind of trial—let **there be no temptation for blame. Judge not that ye be not judged; for with what judgment ye mete to thy fellow men it shall be meted to thee again**.

Let thy yeas be yea and thy nays be nay, in the Lord. For in Him alone ye live and move and have thy being. While for the time there may be shadows that cause doubt and fear, know that the Lord is in His holy temple; and keep ye quiet, calm within, if ye would hear and know His voice as He speaks with thee.

2600-2 F.62 10/8/41

Q. In this present situation what can I do to bring in more harmony? Is this situation chiefly my fault? If so, how can I improve it and where am I to blame? If not my fault, what am I to do about it?

A. *Who* is blameless? Only those that blame no one for aught that is, has been or may be. Only in creating hope, life, understanding, harmony, does one become blameless. For, as ye understand, they that would be loved must show themselves lovely; they that would have friends must *be* a friend to others. For in the manner ye treat others, ye treat thy Lord.

Let that light which has aroused thee be *alive, awakened.*

Condemn no one. And as ye come seeking, know, understand, as ye create same in the lives of others so is it reflected in thine own.

Charity
2603-1   F.67   10/15/41

Q. Should I continue my charity work for the "Friends of Children" organization, or could I render a greater service to humanity elsewhere? If so, where and how?

A. **No greater service may be rendered than that in aiding children. They are the hope of the world.**

In every form where there may be the betterment of opportunities for children with promise, do same.

2697-1   M.48   3/11/42

For the soul's entrance is the manifestation and the expression of the universal consciousness or God. Thus the relationship the entity may bear to that consciousness brings urges, latent and manifested—whether in the realm of the physical consciousness or the realm of the spiritual consciousness.

As a composite of the latent and manifested urges existent, we find:

The entity is one studious in nature; one who loves animals or pets; one rather inclined to be stingy or "close"—according to some associates.

We find that the entity is one rather set in its tenets or beliefs; one that must learn to open the hand to the needy, else he will open the door to the physician.

2981-4   M.34   12/1/43

Q. What charitable work can I do to make me more worthy to my fellow man?

A. It isn't charitable work that's needed! It's yourself that's needed. It is yourself that you need to expend in helping others! Charity doesn't go much farther than the fellow you contact talking about what a big fellow you are in glorifying yourself in an organized work. But serving yourself is quite different—and is that which counts the most.

3063-1   M.56   6/26/43

Think not that, because they may apparently apply only to the mediocre mind, or to those that are of or in a certain faith, that they do not apply to thee. But know that the truth is applicable in every experience of the entity's life, whether as a shoestring vendor or a seller of such, or a director of some great financial institution, or even a leader or ruler over many peoples.

For the same tenet that applies in one is true in the other. For he that would declare, "If I were so and so, how charitable I would be," or "If I were in this or that position what an effort I would make to magnify this or that," only attempts—in saying such—to give others a high opinion of self, and yet is not fooling even himself or anyone else! For if you give not when you have not even sufficient, though you were blessed with many millions, very possibly you would be much more stingy than you are now—and much harder to get along with—though you declare you wouldn't be!

3663-1   M.63   2/16/44

Q. What proportion of net earnings from any endeavors should I give to the Association for Research and Enlightenment, or church?
A. These should be chosen by the entity. For what is to be given in this or that direction for any purpose **shall be prompted by the real heart of the individual**, and not be even a suggestion from others.

Condemnation
295-2   F.27   11/10/30

Q. How can the entity best overcome the loneliness that so often besets her?

A. Fill the life with the interests of others, and not so much of self—or belittle self, or condemn self for the conditions. Fill the life in the interests of others.

Q. Just what does this phrase in the life reading mean, "We find those of the natures taking on that of application of self's abilities to the aid, benefit, of others not *in* such relations will fill, should fill, the present experience to a life worthwhile and the greater development for the entity in the present experience will be found through such channels"? Just what does it mean by, "not *in* such relations"?

A. Just what has been given in this, that there is—has been—too much in the present experience of the condemnation of others and of self. This makes for those conditions as are here outlined. The remedy—as given—**be more interested in the affairs, conditions, of others—but of others that are of the same mental and spiritual inclinations.**

342-2   M.48   5/29/33

And each soul may find that self-condemnation becomes, after all, the hell in which it finds itself in the transition periods.

Hence in the present experience the entity finds much of the commercial field being of interest, especially that as in relationships to the tradings between groups, masses and individuals or groups may be made the more satisfactory to the entity in the present experience . . .

421-5   F.21   10/20/31

In Venus we find (that as the inclination) one with an even disposition. While tempestuous thoughts arise, and the body-mental supersensitive to reactions in others, and the feelings are easily hurt; yet lovable in mien, in manner, and looks and feels towards others as all would do right, even as self would. These are well, and when there arises disappointments in individuals, or in groups, through falseness in any manner, do *not* condemn self or the *weakness* in others. Rather hold fast to that as is set as the *ideal*, and dislike *not* the individual; rather that [which] forces, or *causes*, them to be false with themselves and others.

462-16   M.58   8/10/42

Q. Any other advice or counsel?
A. Keep the mind clear from condemning of self or of others, and we will keep a better physical reaction as well as a mental that will be more constructive in whatever service is chose.

Do have the physical body in better reaction before accepting *any* specific or regular service. For, these are necessary under those existent conditions.

And know, deep in self, the law of the Lord is perfect.

1786-1   F.38   1/11/39

Before that we find the entity was in the English land during those periods when there were the preparations made for the journey of the men into other lands for an ideal; in the defense of that known as the Holy Land.

Those brought for the entity material and mental disturbances; and the differences of opinion that arose between the entity's associates, the entity's companions, brought a great deal of distress.

Hence in the present we find that peoples and their activity constantly become disturbing factors in the entity's experience.

Look, my child, rather to thine own skirts. Keep them clean. **Live towards others as ye would have them live towards thee, and hold *that* rather than any condemning of those who live their *own* life according to that *they* have partaken of—whether for the weal or woe.**

Let thy yeas be yea and thy nays be nay, to be sure; but learn *tolerance! That* is thy lesson to gain in this experience, and with it its sister—not step-sister either—*patience!* Patience, persistence, tolerance! These must be kept in thy activities, as ye did *not* in those experiences as Myra Kingsley.

1786-2   F.39   7/10/39

As has been outlined, first study self. What *do* you desire? Is it selfish, is it only for self; is it only that there may be the gratifying of an emotion, an appetite, a physical desire? or is there not something that is more lasting, something that is desired to be of a *helpful* force for someone else?

Is there really the desire to know love, or to know the experience of someone having an emotion over self? Is it a desire to be itself expended in doing that which may be helpful or constructive? **This *can* be done, but it will require the *losing* of self, as has been indicated, *in* service for others.**

Do not continue to condemn self nor others. The warnings have been in respect these. There are abilities in those fields of activity of story writing. This may be accomplished, if it will go about to do same. But wishing does not do it—application only!

2061-1   F.34   12/12/39

In the present experience, let those activities be such that, though there may come into the experience the separation in the relationships with those who are near and dear, there may be no condemnation in thine own self, or in thine own part, or thy finding fault with any. For, know that if justice had been, or were, or should be demanded of any soul, it would be as if it were not. For He is mindful of His children, ever; and as a loving Father pitieth His children.

So will He, that is the Maker of heaven and earth, He that is the uprising and the downsitting of all mankind, bring to thy life and thy experience that necessary for thy labors are spent in the activity for others, rather than attempting to justify ideas of any moral, physical or mental relationships.

Know that truth and honor need no justification; rather the glorifying of same only is righteousness in the sight of thy Maker.

2117-1   F.31   2/27/40

Remember, there are no shortcuts to mental and spiritual success. It (success) must be labored for, and service rendered.

And in patience and in truth, keep self unspotted from condemnation—from others or from self's own conscience.

For, a soul, an entity, does not enter by chance, but that indeed there may be in the experience of each soul that love, that mercy, that grace which is manifested in the experiences of those who *have learned* the lesson, "Seek ye the Lord while He may be *found!*"

Make His purposes thine own, and *then* all the material, the mental things that go to make a pleasant experience in a material sojourn will come unto thee.

But in patients, in love, in gentleness, in kindness, seek first to show thyself *worthy* of being granted that mercy, that love, which a loving Father-God seeks to manifest in the experience of all who seek His face.

5075-1   F.50   5/8/44

See in self, then, the virtues as well as the faults. Then, magnify the virtues, **minimize the faults.**

Don't condemn self more than you would be condemned by thy Maker. Don't pass over frailties of others because of strength in self, but see thyself as thy abilities and the urges, and know that in Creative Energies, in God, in Christ as God, ye may find strength for the application of thy ideals.

Others, yes, is thy motto. But not others to such an extent or degree as to become so zealous as to forget the first principles. What ye sow, ye reap, unless ye have passed from the carnal or karmic law to the law of grace.

Then know that whatever exists is for a purpose, for He having overcome the world may aid thee in overcoming the world.

5231-1   F.64   6/5/44

In giving the interpretations of the records, there is much from which to choose. Here we would minimize the faults, for so will the Christ if the body, mind and soul will but take Him as a guide. Remember, as that one taken in what men called a fault and the law demanded the life by stoning, yet the Master forgave, so may ye be forgiven.

We would then, as would He give: Magnify the abilities and, as He said, keep those abilities in the home, in the efforts for beautiful homes, that love may reign in the homes of those who are about the entity. Thus may ye, even as Marie [Mary Magdalene?] of old, become a shining light because ye have known how to forgive, because ye have been forgiven.

In interpreting those purposes, those urges, those which are latent and those which are manifested:

There is manifested the desire that the entity itself may yet, may now, be as a helpful influence in the lives and the experiences of others. Not by condemnation, then, but by appreciation of what has been, what are the weaknesses, what are the shortcomings of those who may by the beauty of thy countenance, as well as by the beauty of thy purpose, attract others to you, who themselves have problems.

Hear them, don't condemn them. Thy Lord did not, why will thou? Advise and counsel with them, rather that thy may take hold on the promises of Him, who has given "A new commandment I give you, that ye love one another, even as I have loved you; who would put myself in your place, who will take upon myself all of thy burdens and make thy cross light."

Thus ye may do to many, and in this ye will find joy, yes, and find love hath not passed thee by at all, but that there are the opportunities for being to others what you would have had others be to thee.

5255-1   F.51   6/15/44

Yes, yes, we have the records here of that entity now known as or called [5255], [see 5255] . . .

There are many commendable activities; there are also questionable ones. **While the entity is very secure in itself, that is, as to its ideas, a question might be asked: are the ideals true, are the activities in their relationships to others in keeping wholly with that which may be claimed as an ideal?**

Have ye analyzed the difference between ideas and ideals? **Ideals are set from spiritual purposes, spiritual aspirations, spiritual desires** and there is a pattern in Him who is the way, the truth and the light, and when that pattern is set according to such judgments, we would find there is never condemning of another. Because others do not agree with thee, condemn then not. For with what judgment ye mete, it is measured to thee again. These ye find as thy greater problems in the present in relationships with others. Then analyze first thyself and thy ideals. Not merely as to, "Yes, I believe this," or "Yes, I believe that," but write it down.

What is thy spiritual ideal? Who is the author of same? Do ye apply same mentally? Is that what ye think of people?

Ye are inclined to say harsh things at times, or not harsh but slighting things, and these grow and multiply by being told or by just being exposed to gossip; and it brings difference, it brings confusion, and these are reflected in thine own experience.

5276-1   F.56   6/17/44

Condemn not thyself for any fault that may have been in others, or for thy having made choices that have apparently brought outer appearances of activities in others not good. Did the Master condemn self for the ways among men? rather, "Of myself I can do nothing, only as the spirit of truth and of the Father may work in and through me, may I become one with His purposes with me."

And He, my friend, is the pattern. He is thy Brother, He is thy Lord. In Him ye live and move and have thy being.

As to the activities in the earth, all may not be indicated, but these are those ye may see in the pattern of self, as have been the promptings through the experiences in the earth:

Before this we find the entity was among those who came to the land of the entity's present sojourn for seeking a manner in which they could of themselves worship God according to the dictates of their own consciousness, in the ways and means and manners as their heart dictated, and not as others would prompt.

Thus we find the entity was in the environ of that now known as or called "the city of brotherly love" and the entity was among those who were close in the relationships to those who were in authority. For the entity was the companion or the wife of one Georgia Penn, and was then in the name Cecelia.

In the experience the entity made for unfoldments and yet many of these became, as it were, as narrow as those from which the entity had sought relief. **And yet, as oft found in human experience, that we condemn in others is, to be sure, the reflection of that which is error in one's own self** . . .

Q. What can I do to make up for the blame I feel regarding this?
A. As has been indicated, blame not self. Say, as did the Master on the cross, and let it be blotted away: Remember it not more, even as He, the Father, remembers no more. For remember, He can only forget and forgive as we forgive ourselves, as well as others.
Q. Why do I feel responsible for my sister . . . committing suicide? Would my return to England have prevented this?
A. Not responsible, but these are condemnations, as has been indicated, arising from experiences in the earth; but leave them where thy belong. Let the dead past bury its dead.

Consistency
288-21   F.23   5/27/28

With conditions as come to the physical forces of the body, let the body be consistent in the activities as to exercise mental and physical; as to well-balanced and well-regulated diet; for not well to digress from that as is produced in system for reaction in proper order. Be regular, whether much or little—not eating much once, not eating anything next time, and then over gorging again. Be consistent . . .

Q. In referring to being warned of the same condition—in what way did the body not carry out those other suggestions, so that the conditions, reoccur?

A. That given at the *time* carried out. The consistency not held to. Reoccurrence of the same condition, even more severe in the present—for, as given, there are no activities at present from the liver. This well tended to cause gallstones, and that as has been called appendicitis. Be warned . . .

294-208   M.67   3/14/44

In the mental and spiritual aspects of the body there needs to be kept consistency of the mental and spiritual activities with the physical aspects of the entity's relationships to the efforts thereof, if there would be kept the better balance in the body.

Keep, then, such an activity physically as to rejuvenate, revivify, the respiratory system; as might be indicated with definite periods each morning for a walk in the air, consistently—not spasmodically; a form of exercise as to cause a better activity through the body—and then just keeping in that way of being consistent.

Don't preach, don't act in one direction and then say or do those things in another direction.

Be patient with those who are weak.

Be kind to those who are even ugly.

Be gentle with those activities wherein there is the necessity that ye live consistently, that ye be consistent with that ye would represent among thy fellow men.

For know, the Lord is in His holy temple. If thou hast, as His child, desecrated thy temple—in word, in act, in deed—know that ye alone may make those corrections, and that thy body is the temple of the living God. Act as though it were, and not as if it were a pigpen or a place of garbage for the activities of others.

Then keep thy body, thy mind, wholly in an active service for thy Lord.

903-6   F.26   6/9/28

Q. Should the body be forced to eat at this time when she doesn't desire food?

A. No. Never force *any* issue for the mental and physical well-being for *developing* body. Only keeping that of consistent regulation of thought and activity, for while desire without mental consistency may lead one—when it has borne fruit—into irregularity as respecting physical or mental attitude; hence consistency, regularity.

Q. What exercise should the body take?

A. These are as constant developments for any well-being, well-balanced body. Consistent exercise with conditions as develop. Walking exercise is well. The general conditions well. General social relations well. Yet these must ever be consistent with conditions as they arise.

2509-2   F.48   9/12/43

Not as a condemnation nor yet as a laudation but rather as a warning to the entity—**there must be consistency in self if you would expect consistency in others.** For, it becomes an irrefutable, unchangeable law, with what measure ye mete, or have meted to thy fellow man, with such measure will it be meted to thee again. For, indeed as has been indicated, it is necessary that offenses come, but woe unto him by whom they come. Think not "I am come to destroy the law"—but "I come to fulfill the law; and ye each entity must pay every whit and every farthing."

It is not by might and power but by the little leaven that leaveneth the whole lump. It is line upon line, precept upon precept, here a little and there a little, that each soul seeks and finds it relationship to the Creative Forces or God—so that it may apply same in its own experience with the fellow man ... For, the entity was in the land of the present nativity, where there were those attempts to draw in the people for the rehabilitating of the lands in portions of Ohio, Indiana and Illinois.

The entity was among those peoples that were settlers in the

land, and the entity was graciousness itself in its treatment of
those about the entity, but—too often for the use of the own self.
Thus the entity became a disappointment to many, yet in self was
satisfied with that which it had attained. Here too, should be a
lesson—**never be satisfied but content.** For, he that is satisfied
has ceased to grow. Being content and consistent becomes another experience for an individual.

2573-1   M.33   8/12/41

The virtue of consistency should be nourished, or the lack of
it corrected. For as the entity journeys through life he should
minimize the faults and magnify the virtues; not only in self and
self's relationships to things to conditions and to individuals, but
also minimize the faults and magnify the virtues to the associates.

Thus the halfway mark, or the being temperate in the
pessimism and the optimism would be a lesson for the entity to
attain . . .

As to the activities in the present, and that to which it may
attain, and how:

First, study thyself. For in the study of thine own nature ye
may better fit thyself to know others; ye may better prepare
thyself for directing and guiding others who may be entrusted
in thy care.

Study to show thyself approved unto thy ideal, that ye choose.

Be consistent in all things, for consistency is indeed a jewel.

3175-1   F.42   8/25/43

Mars brings that abundance of energies, activities rather than
anger. Anger, to the entity is a fearful state. Do not let that which
ye fear come upon thee. Replace same rather with patience, con-
stancy and—most of all—consistency. **For, consistency is a gem
which few souls acquire, in the interpretation or understanding in speech or in conversation with others.**

3205-1   M.13   9/10/43

As to the abilities of the entity:

Study self and self's relationship to Creative Forces. Do first things first, though ye intend oft to do such and become negligent. Put this far from thee in thy experiences with others. For, those that are not consistent with self will not be with others.

3503-1   F.44   12/15/43

The entity should begin first with the spiritual self. What are the ideals in the spiritual self? What are the sources of thy hope for a continued consciousness after this material life? For as it may be considered, it isn't all of life just to live, nor all of death just to die, but what is prompting the hope of the future life—spiritually, mentally, materially? Are you as an individual living such a life that would be consistent in producing that ideal in relationship to all concerned in problems that are a part of the experience in the present?

Then, when the life is made consistent with the ideals, we will find health, greater relationships, greater help of every character may be experienced in the body, in the mind of this entity.

Be consistent, then, with self. Be consistent with the ideals.

Then they may be so lived in the experience as to mentally and materially demand or seek such in the relationships with others.

Do this and we will find life becoming more worthwhile—for self, for those with whom the entity comes in contact daily.

By the very living—not by word but by deed also—make life worth living for others.

3605-1   M.31   1/21/44

Hence so plan thy activities that each phase of thy consciousness is stimulated to activity, regularly, and ye will get away from the waiting for changes, or the being very high in ideals one day and because of some little slight ready the next day to "cuss out" the other fellow.

This means consistency, which indeed is a jewel in the experience of any soul-entity.

As to the appearances in the earth, these have been quite varied. While all may not be indicated in the present, these are given as the indications of the latent and manifested urges showing why, in the application of self through experiences, there are those unusual combinations of astrological aspects (so termed) in the entity.

Before this entity was in the land of the present nativity, during the early settlings—when there were varied groups in various sections with certain tenets or truths which they expected or hoped to make predominant in that particular phase of the experiences in the land.

The entity was among those who came in the early periods from Ireland, then in the name of Joseph McArty. The entity was in aid to those who would establish an activity for the church, though the entity in its application among the natives—with the variations that came about—slipped far away from the general tenets set by those in authority.

Hence in the present there are the appearances at times of being very religious, and the feeling that it is very necessary for some people but not so necessary for self—except at times when you have need of same. In this respect there needs to be the exercising of self in consistency. Not merely in thought but in application, so as to keep well-rounded, well-balanced in stimulating physical, mental and spiritual phases of the entity.

4038-1   F.53   4/7/44

Then counsel well with self, as well as with others, but from the principles and tenets of Him who was the way, the truth, and the light. For there is no other name given under heaven whereby men may be saved, and that's from themselves, as well as from the evils that so many individuals think are the cause of other people attempting to gain control politically or financially. Their sources and their principles are one.

In judgment, then, as so often given, study to show thyself

approved unto God. That is presupposing that thy ideals are the law of the Lord; rightly stressing the words of truth and giving due consideration, being all things to all peoples. Put thyself in the other individual's place, and not merely because "I think it is this or I know this is true," but consider. For if mercy and justice were measured by the heavenly Father, as it would be by thyself, would thee be consistent? Consistency is the jewel that most souls need. You cannot be one thing today and something else tomorrow. There must be consistency.

Constructiveness
261-13   M.47   11/22/34

Q. Are there any suggestions or advice further for this body at this time?
A. **In the physical keep the body in those attitudes that make for constructive forces in the body at all times.**
In the mental attitude and the associations and relations, keep those that make not only for the betterment of self but of all the associations—through keeping the spiritual insight as the basis for all activities.
261-25   M.48   10/4/36

Q. Any further advice?
A. Keep optimistic, and keep spiritually balanced. For the sources of mental and material influences must arise, as so oft has been given, from a spiritual import that is *constructive*! **Hence an individual that does not *think* constructively builds barriers to be tumbled over sooner or later.**

270-44   M.55   3/25/40

Q. Do you find my body in as good physical condition as that found before?
A. In some respects, better; in others, not so well. The anxieties and aggravations which have been experienced through the mental forces of the body have naturally tended to upset, and

to give impulses in the physical functions for irritations, where those disturbing conditions have existed heretofore. Thus, some of these show inclinations that are not so well.

There should be more precaution, then, as to keeping a better mental attitude, or a more constructive attitude, even under adversity; and keep the exercises and the eliminations better.

270-47   M.56   4/25/41

Q. Is there any specific advice respecting personal conduct and the mental attitude applicable to my work and relations with my associates that requires special cultivation in that greater confidence and cooperation will be more evident?
A. As indicated, there has been a great improvement since last we had these conditions. We would continue in those lines and in those activities; keeping the constructive attitude as of being a helpful influence in its associations with all its activities and its relations . . .
Q. Will you now outline for my guidance the new order of things that will follow culmination of the present world affairs and the plan that I should adhere to in my relation with associates?
A. As we find, it would not be well even to attempt to outline this in the present conditions. For, conditions will grow more and more extravagant, or there will be those periods when there will be greater anxiety — even at times reaching to those stages of some activity on the border of overanxiety, see?
Thus it will depend upon the final choices and decisions that will be made, as to what new orders will come or what new conditions will arise.
But maintain at all times with the associates, and with all relationships with those with whom the entity comes in contact in the present as well as in the future periods, the attitude of being and remaining in a constructive experience for each and every one. Only as you would that others should do, you should do. Not under the stress and strain attempting to make for the saving of self irrespective of others, but one for all, all for one . . .

Q. Is there any further advice for me at this time?

A. **Keep the mental attitude towards spiritual living as the basis for all mental and material activities; and we will find that which is being sought will be nearer in keeping with creative and corrective influences in the experience in every phase of the life.**

480-19   F.23   7/12/35

Q. Any further advice for my welfare?

A. Keep a constructive, *optimistic* attitude towards the associations, the environs, the surroundings. As has been indicated, the relationships that will arise from the undertakings in the conditions of the body will be aided by those activities, if the precautions are taken that will make such *as* a portion of the *experiences* that make for *bodily* help.

Keep in the attitude, then, of helpfulness, hopefulness; and we will find life and its experiences more and more worthwhile.

Keep the faith of thy fathers in those relationships thou would establish.

494-2   F.Adult   12/5/37

Q. Any other advice for the body?

A. Keep *mentally* in that attitude of *constructive* thinking, ever. **Never allow self to become pessimistic or doubtful, or fearful as to the activities about the body in any form.**

694-2   F.45   10/16/34

. . . To thine own self in these relationships be true, and thou wilt not be false to any—to whom thou shouldest show forth in thine life, thine expression of life, thine activities in the material things, the love even of the Father. *Be* rather, then, in thine associations in friendships, the impersonal; yet with the love of thy fellow man so deep, so high, as to show forth *that* love that passeth understanding. For *rest* rather than in those promises that

He has given, in "A new commandment I give, that ye love one another," and thus *fulfill* the law of love. Love *is* law, law *is* love, to those that love *His* appearing.

From the influences in Mercury we find one of high *mental* application, yet not always has the entity found it in self to easily discern whose end was in the constructive direction. Then, those that proclaim the love of *constructive* thought are those things that may bring in thine mental and in thine spiritual experience the *constructive* experiences in thine moral, thine social, thine commercial life. **For if ye be not founded in grace and mercy to thy fellow man, may thou expect grace and mercy from thy Maker?** For ye are *His* in the earth, and as ye show forth the Lord in thine activity do ye gain understanding as to that which is helpful, that is hopeful, that is peace-giving. **Cry not "Peace, Peace" when thou, thyself, hast not *shown* peace to thy brethren!**

707-2   M.58   2/1/35

Q. In my experience in Rome and Greece, what were "those understandings, tenets, teachings of the man of Galilee"?
A. Walk in the light, even as He is in the light, with thine eye single to the service in the light of Him and His ways. These are the tenets, or as He gave, the first and the great commandment, "Thou shalt love the Lord thy God with *all* thine heart, thine mind, thine soul, and thy neighbor as thyself." And "As ye do it to these, my brethren, ye do it to me. I abide in the Father, ye abide in me, I in the Father, ye in me may be one." These are the tenets, these are the manners that ye present it to thy brethren. These ye heard as the dictates of thy walks among thy brethren. These ye may hold this day; not ever a grudge, not ever an unkind word or thought; these be the fruits of the spirit. "Ye abiding in me may abide in that light that makes the roughest ways but as a way to that peace in Him." For, "Love ye one another."

Contentment
228-3   M.45   1/17/33

A. Keep in that way that is well, regarding the mental, the spiritual and the physical well-being; knowing that the mental is the builder, the *directions* are either from material or spiritual import. Then be *guided* by that that must bring the greater contentment in the well-being at all times.

238-2   F.43   2/13/30

Q. In the association of Mr. Lynch with [238] and her husband [240], what do the forces feel to be the matter and what procedure would the forces suggest?
A. This becomes rather of the personal or individual nature, for in the supervision there comes those of combative influences — **for the *soul* of [238] has grown beyond that of Lynch and to be led by one that is beneath is but to bring those developments that are often contrariwise to the understanding of each, and builds for each that which brings and *breeds* discontent. Being content, is a happy position. Being *satisfied*, is being lost.**

347-2   F.59   6/5/33

The greater an individual, the more content the individual may be. Not as an animal that is satisfied with the body filled, but rather that contentment which is seen in the acts of those that bring joy with the expression of themselves; as a bird in song, a bird in flight, an animal in the care of its young. *That* is contentment; the other rather lethargy.

352-1   F.17   6/9/33

As we have indicated, there are two ways lying before the entity. These may be chosen *best* by self; for the gift of the creative influence is that — in the life, or in material affairs, termed in the lives of each soul — there are the abilities to make self, through the application of will, one with the constructive influences or to turn same to self's own indulgencies.

And those that seek to know self may find the way. Those that find the way become content, and find joy, peace, happiness, even though the way be hard.

Those that look for self-indulgencies, self-interests, without being tempered with the true love as of the Father in life *to* those that seek His way, *these* find those things that make for hardships, strifes, turmoils, even though there are—from the *material* standpoint—abundances of earth's materials, earth's storehouse, in the experience of an entity.

Then, seek Him while He may be found. Build the life in those things that make for constructive influences in the experiences of others; for in so doing will the help come as from the hills of the Lord.

417-1   M.35   9/10/29

We find one that may be controlled by reason, by love, by honor, by those innate desires to accumulate those forces in power—that is, tempered with justice and with love.

In the experiences in the present experience the changing in will has brought much to the entity in the present, and will—with this continued activity—build that which will bring to the entity that satisfaction and contentment that only controlling of self is possible to bring to an entity. Not satisfied that makes of the stillness, or the inactivity, but that contentment of the life well lived, and the justice done to the brother in the best of the entity's abilities.

Depression
5639-2   F.50   7/25/29

Q. How much of my depression is due to the irrational life of my son, [...]?
A. Just as much as the body allows!

Desire
1293-1   F.39   11/17/36

Self-glory, self-exaltation, self-indulgence becometh those influences that become as abominations to the divinity in each soul; and *separate* them from a knowledge of Him. For thou *art* persuaded, for thou *knowest* from thine experience, *nothing* may separate the soul of man from its Maker but desires and lusts!

1703-2   F.51   12/12/38

Q. What was meant in the reading by: " . . . the activity of the mental self . . . producing the plethoric conditions"? Does this refer to difficult situation in the past or to an attitude of mind that I should strive to correct?
A. This rather what might be said to be a combination. That the attitude of mind in the past to conditions, circumstances and surroundings has caused a great deal of disturbance that has been and is a part of the present experience is evidenced. Then, **the attitude of mind should be toward *knowing* that the influences of every force within the experience of an individual are a part of that individual's activity in any given environ or surrounding.**

Then when *any* condition is set wherein there are resentments to conditions such that there is builded the influences or forces to meet or overcome, these become natural problems to the mental self—and find reflection in the activity of same through the physical forces of the body.

As may be a very poor but very definite illustration of same: When there is the approach of the body to an environ from which there is the odor of foods of certain character, there is aroused within the mental self either a desire for the satisfying of the appetite within that direction or there is builded the attitude that it should be put aside because it produces such and such in the system, because Jim, Jane or John said so! and yet the very inner self calls for those influences, *knowing* that within self the body, the mind and soul are a material representation of every influence that is without the self—that may be viewed or become aware of by self.

Then the mind or mental self, or mental body, that is the builder for the physical as well as the directions from the spiritual, should be made to coordinate and cooperate; and *use* and not abuse the knowledge of self!

1754-1   F.20   11/25/38

Do two wrongs make *anything* right? Have ye lived, will ye and do ye live day by day as ye would that men should do to you, do ye even so to them?

This is the law, this is the *ideal*. Not merely idealistic but the Way of Life.

And as in thine abilities, in thine *innate* desire—*none* may be more beautiful in purpose, in the life, in the ability to *give* to others joy, peace, contentment—with all the attributes of the earthly things combined—passion, with all of its material loves, all of its material desires. These ye know well; but unless these be tempered with thine ideal, thy *will* may lead thee in the paths that become troublesome, dark and disagreeable!

Determine then whom ye will serve. That of thine own self that may bring discouragements, despairs? Or Him who hath promised, "My peace I give—not as the world giveth peace, but that which is love, and hope, and kindness, and godliness."

1947-3   F.31   9/4/39

"My Spirit beareth witness with thy spirit as to whether ye be the children of God or not." This becomes, then, that force, that influence for comparisons; as the entity meditates upon its own emotions, its own influences, these become very apparent within itself for comparisons.

Do they bespeak of kindness, gentleness, patience—that threshold upon which godliness appears?

Desire may be godly or ungodly, dependent upon the purpose, the aim, the emotions aroused.

Does it bring love? Does it bring long-suffering? Is it gentle?

Is it kind?

Then, these be the judgments upon which the entity uses those influences upon the lives of others.

Does it relieve the mental anguish, the mental disturbances which arise? Does it bring also healing—of body, of mind, to the individual? Is it healed for constructive force, or for that as well bring pain, sorrow, hate and fear into the experience of others?

These be the judgments upon which the entity makes its choices, as it guides, directs or gives counsel to those who are seeking—seeking—What? That Light—which has become, which is, which ever was the light of the world!

What was that light? The Spirit of God moved, and there *was* light! That Light came—the light of men—yea, dwelt among men as *mind* with the ability to choose, the ability to abstain, the ability to put away desire, hate, fear, and to put on the whole armor. All of these are attributes then of those influences and forces which are a part of the entity's experience.

And as these are applied, so may the entity come to apply its psychic abilities, its love, its desire, its hopes, *spiritualized* in self-effacement by placing God's *glory*, God's *love*, in the place of self; bringing hope, *hope* and *faith* in the minds and hearts, the lives of others.

This is the mission of the entity in this experience; fulfilling much of that sought after, much of that at times lost in self-desire. But often seeking, knowing, applying, ye become closer and closer in an at-onement with Him.

These are the purposes, these are the desires, these are the manners in which the mental may be applied for the soul and spiritual development; and in the manner, "As ye do it to the least of these, thy brethren, ye do it unto me," saith the Lord.

2269-1   F.31   5/31/40

Do ye indeed know what jealousy and hate breed? Do ye know what longings and desires create, that are only gratifying the emotions of the body? and how they become as hangers-on in the form of habits that may undermine?

Then, only hope and faith, and kindness, and gentleness, brotherly love and patience, beget that strength, that harmony, that peace
which is of the everlasting nature as promised in Him.

2725-1   F.36   5/14/25

... Service to others the greatest service to the Creator. The desire to seek the greater forces will gradually bring, draw, make,
accomplish the desired end in the same manner as pennies accumulated finally reach to the desired amount for any purchase.
Apply all rules pertaining to life to that.

3234-1   F.24   9/23/43

Here, in the present environ, was the entity's appearance in the
earth before this—one who had taken the vows and found love
of the material things caused the entity to break those vows of
celibacy. This brought to the entity material joys, and yet the
entity feared throughout the experience that these were for self
rather than toward that purpose which had been determined by
the entity.

Know, all the desires of the body have their place in thy experience. These are to be used and not abused. All things are holy
unto the Lord, that He has given to man as appetites or physical
desires, yet these are to be used to the glory of God and not in
that direction of selfishness alone.

Let this be rather the tenet of the mind, of the soul, of the
body: Success must be to the glory of God rather than to the
gratifying of any appetite, of any desire, of fame or fortune.
Know that fame and fortune must be the result of thy seeking in
His paths first, and then all will be lighted along the way.

3795-1   F.   Adult   4/2/31

... *Desires* are good, are desires controlled by the best *interests*
for the body mentally and physically. Not merely those as satisfy
the desires of the body physical, but those desires that build for

a continuity of life's forces within an individual. Then, with the changes, has come an awakening of abilities within the body. These, as we find, make for desires—or rather wishes—that there might be some great change come into the life. These are well, for such changes may *come*—will the body but apply those abilities in whatsoever direction the surroundings, the time, the place, gives the opportunity for the application of those things known within self, that makes for making life, making surroundings, a little more pleasant, a little more harmonious, a little more of those that make for a regeneration within; not giving away to desires that satisfy for the moment, not allowing self to become in any manner selfish with self, self's abilities—or, as may be better put, *preferring* another—or others—before self . . . . . . Not as done *for* the *reward*; rather let thine heart, thine mind, thine *being*, be opened as with the love that passeth all understanding; remembering as it was said of old, "Though I have faith that removes mountains, though I speak with the tongues of angels, though I may conquer even the world and have not *that* love, it is *nothing*," for it becomes as an emptiness that *cannot* be filled—but with each day, each hour, so lived as an act that the self would present before the throne of grace, and *all* power is given to those who *do* in *this* manner His biddings, and the *Spirit* abideth ever! Only thine self may turn thy face from *His* face. Only thine self may make a shadow upon His abiding Spirit; for in *His* likeness, in *His* image, are we *all* made. Turning as upon thine own self casts the shadow.

5563-1   F. Adult   4/24/30

Put self rather, then, in the hands, in the mind, of the *Divine* from within, and not attempting, not *trying* to be good, to be kind, to be thoughtful—but just *be,* and *consecrate* self to the service of others. This peace, this quietness that will come within self from such, will find a ready answer in the mind, in the heart, in the life, in the expression of those—every one—whom the body contacts. *This* **is** *living* **consecration, and not attempting to be moral for moral's sake;** not attempting to be good that good may come, but be good that there may be that peace, that understanding, that only comes from putting self in the hands of the Divine. study, then, portions—*any* portion—of the words of Him that gave that, "That ye ask in my name, *believing*, that shall ye have within yourself." Do not, then, in asking, make conditions—but surrender self unconditionally into the hands of the Divine from within, and that from within shall answer—even as was said, "My spirit beareth witness with your spirit that ye are called the sons, the daughters, of the *living* God," for in Him only is that peace, and the blessings of those whom the body *contacts* will bring the greater joy, the greater happiness. Happiness, then, is not a thing set apart from self, but the conditions with which one approaches that in hand to be *done*! for when one considers that the position of self is hard to bear, is not as is desired, the desire of the heart often maketh one *afraid* —unless that desire is ever in that attitude of *"Use me*, O God, as I am,: for the I AM is ready, willing, to make *my* will *one* with *Thy will*—"Though He slay me, though He bruise me in mine own selfish or unseen way; yet will I trust Him day by day," and He will *not* forsake thee; neither will He allow thee to be afraid; for He will raise thee up, and He understands all the hardships, the *little* things, the separations, the variations in the surroundings—but *trust* Him!

In this manner may the body, the mental body, the physical body, allow the spirit of Truth, peace, joy, understanding, come in and make for self, for those dependent upon self, mentally and physically, whole and strong—and able and capable of meeting every issue of *every* day . . .

5752-3   11/8/33

How to determine that which is good and that which is evil?

In the application does the seeker find that which answers to that *it* has set as *its* ideal, that *it* may worship, that *it* may become one with in its consciousness, in its sphere.

What separated spirit from its first cause, or [what] causes good and evil?

Desire! *Desire*!

Hence Desire is the opposite of Will. Will and Desire, one with the Creative Forces of Good, brings all its influence in the realm of activity that makes for that which is constructive in the experience of the soul, the mind, the body, one with the spirit of truth.

Disappointment
3416-1   F.39   11/23/43

Q. Please give me my life seal and its interpretation.
A. Let's make this later, not here. These are to be builded more in self than as an inspiration. For as indicated, many of the experiences have come as disappointments. Let's not remind the entity of disappointments. For as He forgives, He forgets. So must ye. Thy memories are well—keep them, for you will forget the hardships and remember the beauties of same.

4037-1   M.36   4/6/44

Then physically apply the necessary energies to revivify, to replenish the energies, the energy-supplying efforts, so that even from the structural portions of body there may be the rebuilding or supplying from that assimilated in physical digestion, the red blood cellular forces to overcome the physical deficiencies and those tendencies of the energies of the body to be destroyed within the own physical self.

We being first then with the mental attitude. Do the first things first. Begin by the closer study within self of self, as related to the universal consciousness or God. The manifestations indicated in His word, then, must be the basis for this relighting, this reviving, this replenishing of the attitudes of the mind and of the spiritual self from those injuries, those hurts, those disappointments.

Let's begin like this: First, **don't be overanxious.** Know that it is within self and that what may be supplied by mechanical means is only the means to an end, and the good that may arise from same is only that this form of application may attune the body to that which may gain in its own mental self, by a study, by an analysis of the relation of self to the universal consciousness or God.

Begin, then, here: Read Exodus 19:5, then the whole 30th chapter of Deuteronomy. Then turn to Romans, read the whole book of Romans; not analyzing but rather knowing that each of these portions refers to self. These are the activities within self. Then begin with St. John 14, 15, 16, 17. Know these almost by heart, but rather as they apply to self, as they each refer to self. For here are promises. They apply to this body as an individual. For the very fact that ye are conscious of yourself should be the assurance that He, the Father-God, is mindful of thee as an individual entity and that ye have work to do. He is depending upon thee for the knowledge, for the glorifying, for the opportunity to glorify Himself through thee. Do this first.

4353-3   F.20   11/12/24

In the mental and spiritual, we find the body well developed in every way. There is in the mental forces those conditions that have brought strain in the mental activity through that of distress or disappointment. In this the body should exercise the mental and the physical to the manner that will give of the best to the work in hand, for this will be found to be both remunerative and give the advancement necessary to make the income from such labors more than sufficient for the needs, and will lead to the success of the entity. While the strain on the body, and the temperament in mental, are such as to work hardships on the mental and spiritual, the relaxing through physical, as outlined, will give much to developing in mental and spiritual forces.

262-17   4/17/32

Q. [288]: Are my attempts at meditation accomplishing anything outside myself?
A. These are but questionings of self, and questionings of the promises are as given!

Might be termed lack of faith in self or the promise! **For each thought, each atom, has its own weight as is expended in whatever direction it *may* be guided by the thought of self!**

To be sure, it *accomplishes*, then, that in self and that outside of self. He that doubteth, then—doubteth self, doubteth Him!

Doubt
262-18   5/1/32

Q. [404]: Does understanding come any with experience?
A. Understanding comes with application. Application may be experience mental or physical, or spiritual. With the ideal that is set before self there comes the awakening. As to whether this is shaken by doubts or fears, or there is the inroads of a doubt that makes for muddying of thine experience, this then makes for a less understanding.

279-4   M.31   7/14/31

In that as has been *builded* in the present experience of the entity in this relationship, as to those influences, those urges, there have come periods when discouragements and those things of secular nature have made doubts and fears arise in the experience of the entity. The doubt has mostly been of self, rather than of thine neighbor, of thine brother, of thine stranger. These come from that urge as is seen in those influences, that when doubts arise, if the entity will look *upon* those troublesome times of a *neighbor*, rather than upon self, *strength* comes from such vision. Never pity self, nor censure self. Rather be *strong* in the weakness of those that give strength. Rather give courage to the disheartened, and *strength* comes from that as has been builded by the entity. **Be not *overcome* of evil, but *overcome* evil with *good*, with deeds of kindness, a cheery word, a smile, a slap on the shoulder. An encouraging word to the faltering gives strength not only to him who falters but aids *self* the more.**

281-3   Glad Helpers Group   12/3/31

Q. In healing is it not paramount to have the body in perfect physical condition?

A. One must raise self to that consciousness of a physical perfection in spirit, to give the proper attitude or physical perfection in spirit, to give the proper attitude or concept to another. *Doubt* never *accomplished* anything!

282-5   M.27   3/22/33

Q. What are the faults or sinful habits of the body-mind?
A. Doubt. Unstable. Not that the purposes, the aims, the desires are lacking; but, the spirit is willing—the flesh mind is weak.
Q. Give suggestions for overcoming these.
A. None better than choosing an hour, an half hour, a twenty minutes of meditation, and seeking to be shown the way. Not just *any* way, but *His* way.

Drudgery
315-9   M.36   9/6/43

Q. What can I do here to make for a more harmonious condition?
A. Just daily application. Do not let it become a drudge or a drag. Be exercised or interested, and in the application use the experiences to enable thee to be of greater service to thy fellow man.

1844-3   M.22   4/30/41

Q. Is the work I do hindering the cure of my eyesight?
A. Not a hindrance; but *do* be reminded to keep the attitude constructive.

For, to any soul, to this particular soul—if the activity is looked upon as a drudge, or as an affliction of any kind, it becomes harmful and detrimental, and aggravating to any physical or mental influence in the body. Remember that . . .

Duty
1532-1   F.18   2/10/38

Duty is well, but the lack of love influence may ofttimes make for misunderstanding. Cultivate rather that in thy experience with duty; not as duty alone but let thy duties always be as *opportunities* for the expressing or manifesting of that as may be chosen as thy ideal.

Have thy ideal, yes—in the material , in the social, in the economic; but above all in the spiritual. For unless all of these—while they are one—are founded upon the spiritual, they will turn upon thee. This indeed is what is meant by that given, "What profit it a man if he gain the whole world and lose his own soul?" or what profit a man who lays up treasures where moth and rust do corrupt, and where thieves break through and steal?

Rather lay up the treasures in the heart, the love, the spiritual things. For these bring the harmony and peace in the experience of the individual that may become the stay, and that upon which one may rest with when the storms of life come about that are in the experience of all.

Egotism
1362-1   M.48   4/27/37

Hence the greater friendships that have in the present experience been a part of the entity's activity, where they have turned—or the entity turned from those associations, have brought greater disturbances.

The loves, the activities in the social life, the activities in the marital life, make for disturbing forces. Duties of either portion of such experience seem to be lost sight of in the moment of *self-will*, self-expression!

Know, self is the only excuse. **Self is the only sin; that is, selfishness**—and all the others are just a modification of that expression of the ego. But so close is the ego, the I Am, to the *great* I AM, THAT I AM, that the confusions of duty and privilege and opportunity become so enmeshed in the experience of the entity.

1391-1   F.62   6/22/37

Only those who become distorted, disturbed, and attempt to express or manifest their own ego, become the more confused—in not having their own way.

2834-1   M.36   10/27/42

As to the abilities of the entity in the present then—these depend upon the ideals chosen. The power, the mind, the might lies within thine own self. Ye *have* been blessed, ye may be again—in thy judgments.

Let not self—as an egotist, or for selfish purposes of any of those things that undermine principle—put thee in the position of neglecting thy opportunities to do good.

Have not only thy ideal materially but thy ideal spiritually, thy ideal mentally.

2987-1   F.33   5/3/43

. . . The ego of self may destroy that which may come to fruition, just as a character of parasite of the mind may destroy the character and abilities of the entity—as indicated in the seal . . .

Learn and practice, first, patience, long-suffering, gentleness, kindness. As ye manifest these, thy are measured back to thee. This is an unchangeable law. For it is spiritual, mental and material—but done because of the seeking only for material, only for mental, must of itself bring confusion. For, know, it is well spoken, "The Lord thy God is *one.*" And it is in Him ye live, ye move, ye have thy being. **The body is the temple of the living God. Thine ego worships there, or at some other shrine. And who possesses thee, when thou art absent from thine own temple—in mind or in spirit?**

3018-1   M.34   5/21/43

The entity because of his indecisions at times allows others to take advantage of him.

The entity must learn to be self-assertive; not egotistical but self-assertive—from a knowledge of the relationship of self with the material world.

3268-1   F.53   10/6/43

There are the abilities also to interest self in the welfare of others and to make the welfare of others a contributing cause to the welfare of a community, county, town or city, or even a state.

Thus the abilities of the entity run in those lines of creative influence as may be seen from Mercury, or there are the high mental abilities of the entity. Keep these ever attuned with the Divine, and put stresses or emphasis on the spiritual as well as the mental attainments. For, knowledge without judgment may easily become sin. **Understanding without spirituality may too soon become egotism.**

Envy
1759-1   M.41   12/14/38

For this experience is for thy own holiness, if ye will but look to Him. For God hath not willed that any soul should be in shame, in discouragement, bound with the fetters of circumstance or of obligation, but would have thee *free*—as He hath given thee thine *own* will—yea, thine own soul, and said, "If ye will be my son, I will be thy God."

Hast thou drawn away? Hast thou neglected thy sonship, thy kinship with thy Maker?

Have ye looked upon the circumstances of others and envied them, or coveted their position or their place? Then, know ye have brought condemnation to thine own self!

Face the light of truth, as is set in Him, and the shadows of doubt and fear, of disappointments and sorrow, will fall far, far behind! For ye will enter into that peace as He hath promised, "If ye will ask, if ye will live in me, I will come and abide with thee."

Exhibitionism
3343-1   M.36   11/1/43

Q. Why do I possess a certain tendency toward physical exhibitionism, and how can it be most effectively subdued?
A. As just indicated. Find the spirit within self. For, as indicated, so oft, think not who will descend from heaven and bring a message, or who will come from over the sea that ye may hear and know. For lo, He is within thine own soul, thine own conscience. Thus does the Master give, "I stand at the door and knock. Open—I and the Father—will enter and abide with thee." He meant it! Would you entertain Him? Then live it

Extremism
1009-4   M.73   8/27/36

In the astrological aspects we find Uranus becoming that making for an extremist in the very activities, and only as the entity has applied self in keeping the self in check in these directions has it prevented the entity from running to the extremes in almost every form of experience; whether in relationships of those of the opposite sex or whether in the activities as related to material gains, or whether in those fields of the preservation even of its own health. These have all been as influences, the tendencies for extremes.

1885-2   M.32   3/26/40

For, as the extremes are so a portion of the entity's experience, know that all phases of human relationships, human endeavors, must be taken into consideration. **And do not become the extremist, as any well-rounded individual may, by allowing self to be drawn off in some particular emotion, some particular activity.**

2449-1   M.60   2/10/41

Yes, forgiveness and karma may at times appear to be extremes;

and yet know that *only* in Him—the Christ—do extremes meet. But that each soul may know, and not lose the way, these *are* experiences—in the meeting of such—as may be borne or understood, or even comprehended, in and with His presence, His purpose, His love.

2880-1   F.56   1/12/43

Q. Considering my intense desire for a constructive use of my knowledge of esoteric astrology in the present, please instruct me as to its purpose and significance in my life; by best procedure in its utilization in my own development and the service and enlightenment of others.
A. Study that as given, in the light, in the life of Him who is the life, the way, the truth, the resurrection. Know, in that manner ye may better apply the understanding to those ye aid, to become a practical everyday experience. For, it is so easy and yet so hard. Know, in Him all extremes meet. For He was, He is, the Creator, the Maker of all that is manifested materially. He came into and unto His own, they received Him not; yet to as many as received Him gave He power to become the children of God. Receive Him, as ye promised Him to others.

4374-1   F.47   12/30/43

. . . As we find, there are tendencies existent regarding which precautions should be taken and corrections made; else the body will find that there may become very serious disturbances.

Yet if the body becomes so health-conscious or so addicted to routines for this or that, it will be just as serious as if the body did little or nothing about it except try to carry on with its work.

Hence there is the need for the mental body, first, to keep itself well balanced. It is well and good to consider the material things and experiences, yet these should not be put first and foremost. Just as self and the physical conditions about the body should not be considered to the exclusion of other abilities, other

duties and obligations that the body has and should have, and
should assume — for many.

Attitudes and Emotions
Part II
Faith
137-12   M.26   1/12/25

Q. How has the body not applied himself, so as to bring about
the results as have just been given?
A. In the lack of the faith in self. Faith, that evidence of that which
manifests in the inner self, through the subconscious knowledge
of those correlated conditions between the conscious and subconscious, acted upon by the superconscious. The application must be
made through the self, and can only be understood by that indwell-
ing answer from within the entity. This can be applied. Apply same.

262-12   2/21/32

Q. How may I increase my faith?
A. Use that thou hast in hand, has been the command from
the beginning, will be unto the end, as to how to increase faith.
**Faith, the substance of things hoped for, evidences of things
unseen. Using that known brings those attunements, those
emoluments in every form, that makes for *Creative* Forces in
themselves — which is, must be, the basis of faith.**

262-18   5/1/32

Q. Please define spiritual faith.
A. **The application of that that is awakened by the spirit within
self.**

281-10   Glad Helpers Group   8/17/32

Q. [993]: Just what method should I use in healing?
A. As has been given, and as has been the experience of self, in

raising the consciousness — in the silence — of those that the body or self would aid, even as it is done in self. As the *experiences* have been, so does the confidence grow in self in that direction. **Confidence, then, is of the material or of the physical sense — while** *faith* **is an attribute of the soul and spiritual body.**

350-1   F.55   6/7/33

The entity then was a daughter of a minister, the name being Wenchelcer.

In the experience the entity thought much, studied much. While the sojourn was not counted in years of great length, the happenings about the entity, the environs of the ecclesiastical or theological terms, and the experiences that brought the attention of many to the ears or to the consciousness *through* the hearing, through the visioning of the entity, brought many experiences — and the entity lost faith, lost confidence (There's a great deal of difference between faith and confidence!) in those about the entity; not as to the abilities of many, yet in the present experience the entity has the ability to be helpful to many that would gain an understanding for themselves of that which *is* helpful, that which *is* questionable, and that which *must* be let alone. **In this direction may the entity give much to others, yet the entity must ground self in an ideal that will not be broken — even as self in that experience.**

459-1   F.33   12/28/29

Q. Please advise body as to her physical attention and welfare.
A. Those are very good. **Keep thine mind attuned to the calls of the Divine within. Keep the body physically fit through the proper exercises — physical and mental — lending most of self's energies to another, and to others, rather than saving self in that,** that would be — he must first be given; for he that seeks the Lord must believe that He is, would they find Him; for one doubting has already builded that barrier that prevents the proper understanding, whether as to physical, mental or spiritu-

al attributes, or spiritual aid, or mental aid, or physical aid; for
that in faith sought for shall be thine, even as was given, "Be my
people and I will be your God . . . "

518-2   F.25   8/13/35

Not in selfishness, not in grudge, not in wrath; not in *any* of those
things that make for the separation of the *I AM* from the Creative
Forces, or Energy, or God. **But the simpleness, the gentleness,
the humbleness, the faithfulness, the long-suffering, *patience!***
These be the attributes and those things which the soul takes
cognizance of in its walks and activities before men. Not to be
seen of men, but that the love may be manifested as the Father
has shown through the Son and in the earth day by day. Thus
He keeps the bounty, thus He keeps the conditions such that the
individual soul may—if it will but meet or look within—find
indeed *His* Presence abiding ever.

The soul, the individual that purposely, intentionally, turns the
back upon these things, choosing the satisfying of the own self's
desire, then has turned the back upon the living God.

Not that there is not to be joy, pleasure, and those things that
maketh not afraid in the experience of every soul. **But the joy in
service, the joy in labor for the fellow man, the joy in giving of
self that those through thy feeble efforts may have put before
them, may become aware in their consciousness,** that *thou* hast
been with, that *thou* hast taken into thine own bosom of the law
of the Lord; and that ye walk daily with Him.

5079-1   F.48   5/8/44

For if ye have not faith in others, how can ye have faith in
God? If ye have not faith in God, how can ye find it in thyself?
Keep sweet, keep true, keep earnest!

5224-1   M.47   6/12/44

As we find, there are disturbances which are preventing the

better physical functioning of the body. These are of rather a complex nature, as some disturbances have been of such long standing as to have become constitutional. Yet these, even in the present, might be helped to a great extent. While it would require patience, persistence and at times it would become rather as something to reckon with, because of the necessity of changing some of the activities to conform to the necessary changes to be brought about, we find that with patience, with persistence, **with faith, many changes can be wrought for this body.**

5326-1   F.23   7/5/44

Q. Are the nerves of motivation dead?

A. If they are, may they not be renewed? **Isn't the body renewed at least once every seven years? Who is to renew it? Who is the giver of life?** By pure coordination, pure faith, pure desire to be what God would have thee be. Ye have much work to do in this material plane. Don't become impatient with self, with others. Know ye are indeed the Lord's only as ye fulfill. His commandments. Read Psalms 119 under the section Tau. Also St. John 14, especially 1st, 2nd, 3rd, 4th, 5th, 6th, 7th, 8th verses and then those latter portions of the 15th chapter. Apply them to self.

Q. Will I be able to walk on my leg by October?

A. **Ye may be able to walk on it tomorrow if ye have sufficient faith, but remember the law of the Lord is perfect; time, space and patience are as necessary attributes of the soul, if it would be one with God, as is body, mind and soul, or Father, Son and Holy Spirit.** They are one and yet remember as He gave: Time is not yet complete, time is not yet at hand, why? the laws are set, love can only remove same. Not that ye are to love other than as he hath loved thee. For He hath not willed that any soul should perish, He will not withhold any good thing from those who love His coming; not their own desire, not those who tell Him how, when and where they must be healed or the way they'll be healed. Seek! For were the lepers who went to Jesus healed as the leper who went to Elijah? Who did the healing? Who would you have do it in thee?

5369-2   M.63   7/19/44

As we find, much might be given as to the characteristics of its abilities in this experience. Yet, add little to these if you would keep in the way that is pleasing to thy Maker. For the entity is one who had used its abilities and its opportunities to offer, to induce, to direct its fellow man in the way that leadeth to a more perfect understanding of the purposes of the experiences of an entity in the material world. That there have been many problems and many questionings is true; yet when the entity has allowed or does allow itself to meditate upon the principles of the prompting which come from its study, its application of the law of the Lord which is manifested in the percepts, the commandments, the psalms and the promises of Jesus, little has been the fear of what the man-force has to offer as to disturbing factors in the earth.

Then, as would be given, keep that faith. Keep the percepts which are the promptings. For these are in keeping with not only the tenets of the entity, but of the tenets of the Book itself. For the law of the Lord is perfect, converting the soul, and the greater the stress, the greater the impress of the purpose upon the life of the Master, greater may be the joys which are found.

Do not let those things which may not in the present be understood weary thy soul, but know that sometime, somewhere, you, too, will understand. Keep the faith.

5749-6   4/5/36

Each soul comes to stand as He before that throne of his Maker, with the deeds that have been done in the body, in the mind, presenting the body-spiritual before that throne of mercy, before that throne of the Maker, the Creator, the God.

Yet as He, the Father, hath given to each of you, "I have given my angels charge concerning thee, and they shall bear thee up, and thou shalt not know corruption."

This He demonstrated in the experience of thy Brother, thy Savior, thy Jesus, thy Christ; that would come and dwell in the hearts and lives of you all—if you will but let Him, if you will but invite Him, if you will but open thy own heart, each of you, that He may enter and abide with you.

Hence when those of His loved ones and those of his brethren came on that glad morning when the tidings had come to them, those that stood guard heard a fearful noise and saw a light, and — "the stone has been rolled away!" Then they entered into the garden, and there Mary first saw her *risen* Lord. Then came they of His brethren with the faithful women, those that loved His mother, those that were her companions in sorrow, those that were making preparations that the law might be kept that even there might be no desecration of the ground about His tomb. They, too of His friends, His loved ones, His brethren, saw the angels.

How, why, took they on form? **That there might be implanted into their hearts and soul that *fulfillment* of those promises.**

What separates ye from seeing the glory even of Him that walks with thee oft in the touch of a loving hand, in the voice of those that would comfort and cheer? For He, thy Christ, is oft with thee.

Doubt, fear, unbelief; fear that thou art not worthy!

Open thine eyes and behold the glory, even of thy Christ present here, now, in thy midst! even as He appeared to them on that day!

What meaneth the story of Christ, of His resurrection, of the man Jesus that walked in Galilee, without that resurrection morn?

Little, more than that of the man thou thinkest so little of, that though his body-physical touched the bones of Elisha he walked again among men!

Dost thou believe that He has risen? How spoke Thomas? "Until I see, until I have put my hand in his side where I saw water and blood gush forth, until I have handled his body, I will *not* believe."

Ye, too, oft doubt; ye, too, oft fear. Yet He is surely with thee. And when ye at this glad season rededicate thy life, thy body, thy mind to His service, ye — too — may know, as they, that He *lives* — and is at the right hand of God to make intercession for *you*—if ye will believe; if ye will believe that He is, ye may experience. For as many as have named the Name, and that do unto their brethren the deeds that bring to them (to you) that closeness, oneness of purpose with Him, may know—ye too—in body in mind, that He *lives today*, and will come and receive you unto Himself, that where He is there ye may be also.

Crucify Him not in thy mind nor in thy bodily activities. Be not overcome by those things that are of the earth-earthy. Rather clothe thy body, thy mind, with the thoughts, the deeds, the privileges that His suffering as a man brought to thee, that He indeed might be the first of those that slept, the first of those that came in the flesh, that passed through all those periods of preparation in the flesh, even as thou.

But if you would put on Him, ye must claim His promises as thine own. And how canst thou claim them unless ye in thine own knowledge, thine own consciousness, *have* done—do do from day to day—that thy heart has gold and does tell thee is in keeping with what He has promised?

For thy Christ, thy Lord, thy Jesus, is nigh unto thee—just now!

Fear
518-2   F.25   8/13/35

Q. What phase of music should I study in order to derive the most benefit?

A. **That more of the nature which to thine own inner self creates *harmonious* vibrations in the experiences of self and those about thee. That partaking of the rimes [rhymes?], the lullabies, the pastoral scenes; which make for such harmonious forces, bring quiet, cheer, hope, and casting out fear.**

578-3   F.21   8/14/34

Q. What can I do to relieve myself of the feeling in the dark of something near, which prevents normal sleep?

A. Surround self in thought with that which may be nearer in every activity that can only be helpful, sustaining; maintaining such an attitude, through the mental and imaginative forces will overcome these conditions.

601-11   F.50   1/17/36

Q. Please give advice as to mental outlook and mental attitudes as referred to in physical check reading given Nov. 22, 1935.
A. This has been discussed here. Again may it be amplified only in this:
Let the law of the *Lord*, as *thou knowest* it in thine heart, *be* the *rule* of *thy* life—and thy dealings with thy fellow man! And ye will find that the growth of the mind-spiritual, of the mind-mental, of the body-physical, will open the way for thee, day by day.

For, as those laws that become as but watchwords to many on the tower, there is a whole day's work before thee each day, with all its glorious opportunities of seeing the glory of the Lord manifested by thine own acts!

Yet if that which confronts thee makes for discouragement, harshness of words, lack of enthusiasm, or those things that make for doubts or fears, the opportunity has turned its back—and what *is* the outlook? Doubt and fear!

Study, then to show thyself approved, *each day! Do what* **thou** *knowest* **to do, to be aright! Then** *leave it alone! God* giveth the *increase! Thy* worry, *thy* anxiety, only will produce disorder in thine *own* mind!

For the application in self, the *try*, the effort, the energy expended in the proper direction, is all that is required of *thee*. God giveth the increase.

1175-1   F.61   5/18/36

Q. How may I develop a spiritual consciousness, so as to make emotionally mine the belief that the so-called dead are alive; that my loved ones are near, loving me and ready to help me?
A. As has been given, know thy Ideal, in what thou hast believed; and then act in that manner, ministering to others. **For perfect love casteth out fear, and fear can only be from the material**

things that soon must fade away.

And thus hold to the higher thought of *eternity*. For life is a *continual* experience. And thy loved ones, yea those thou hast loved. **For what draweth thee nigh to others, to do a kindly deed; to pass a kindly word to those that are disconsolate, those that are in sorrow?** It makes for a bond of sympathy, a bond of love that surpasseth all joy of an earthly nature.

1189-1   F.22   4/28/36

Yet if the entity will hold to the ideal in the present this fear may be eliminated. Know that those forces that arise from self as a manifestation alone of self bring fear; but the expression, the living of those forces that motivate the acts in those periods that are being depicted or expressed by the entity, by the self, rises above those things that would make afraid.

1201-1   M.54   6/29/36

Hence in the experience of the entity in the present there has ever been the urge—which has been as a key to the whole of the entity's experience—to remain free from any ism, cism, sect or influence that makes for *binding* the entity in a direction of activity to *free souls* from fear!! For fear is—as it ever has been—that influence that opposes will, and yet fear is only of the moment while will is of eternity. **Hence fear takes hold upon the emotions, while will is deeper-seated into the soul, into the warp and woof of the very being of an *entity* in its entirety;** finding expression to be sure in the lowest of the emotions, yet is prompted by the Creative Force itself.

Hold fast to that as thou didst experience as a development in those experiences where not only physical aid, not only economic independence in relationships to experiences was brought, but the activities were such that made for *freedom—freedom—*of mind, of soul, to seek, to know, to experience its relationships to its Creator, its mate, its part of itself. For the Creative Forces are more even than companionship; for the heritage of each soul is to know itself to be itself yet one with that Creative Force . . . For the earth *is* the Lord's and the fullness thereof, and they that partake of its glories for their own self-gratification become liars and thieves and murderers in purpose. But to use same for the glorification of the Creator is the purpose.

These the entity used, misused; yet those things are being met in thine experience. **But *hold fast* to that thou knowest in thine inner self; *freedom* from those things that maketh afraid!** . . .

Q. Into what specific fields of activity should I now direct my efforts?

A. As there are the beginnings of those of science, of philosophy, to seek for the knowledge of the true relationships to the soul, then in those activities that may aid those seekers—whether they be the laymen or whether they be the great or those that would be great but aren't. Aid them in their seeking; remaining free in self as in the advice to those, not becoming hidebound or so set in a line that the knowledge of those things that are making for fear in the experiences of those about you is lost sight of.

In such a field may the greatest help, the greatest blessings to self and the greater help to others come.

Q. Should I go back to medical practice?

A. Not as to medicine alone. For again would you take upon the whole of thy experience that which would make thee condemn thyself day by day?

The *earth* is the Lord's. **Be not afraid. If you would create that in the minds of others, then don't act like it yourself! Be** *free!*

5030-1   F. 50   4/16/44

In analyzing and interpreting the records indicated from the entity's experiences in the earth, as well as urges arising from sojourns in realms of consciousness or other phases of consciousness, we find an entity well gifted in many things, yet subject to much of that which is interpreted in self as fear. Yet the entity rarely acknowledges such. **Remember through faith, love, kindness, patience, long-suffering, one may cast out fear.**

If this entity, in this particular sojourn, would make advancements materially, mentally, spiritually, it must first apply in self that which will wholly cast out fear; fear of others, fear of influences, fear of what may come to pass. For if the entity comes to that consciousness which is a part of the universal consciousness, that ye abide—in body, mind and purpose—as one with the Creative Forces, ye are at peace with the world and have nothing to fear. For God will not allow any soul to be tempted beyond that it is able to bear—if the soul puts its whole trust in the Creative Forces manifested in the Christ Consciousness ...

The entity should use these abilities rather as an investigator than as one would apply such. Rather let the universal consciousness and its trust and faith, hope and desire in same be the activity; let the results come of themselves ...

... **Know what ye believe and know who is the author of thy beliefs; not just because you have been taught this or that by any man.** They can only bring to your mind that already contained and all those influences which may add to or take from, according to what spirit or truth ye entertain. For truth maketh thee not afraid. Truth is truth everywhere the same, under every circumstance. It is creative. For light, the Christ, Jesus is the truth, is the perfect way. They who climb up some other way are thieves and robbers to their own better selves.

Then know what ye believe and the author of it. Know that He is able to keep that ye commit unto Him. So, walk and talk oft with Him. For thy body indeed is the Temple of the living God. For He hath promised to meet thee, in humbleness, in love, in patience, in kindness. Thus may all fear be cast out.

Astrological urges have come to mean little, only that they are as urges. **But no urge surpasses the will of self in its relationship to Creative Forces.**

That thou art conscious of being thyself [5030] now, should be evidence to thee that the First Cause, God, is mindful of thee and hath given thee an opportunity to be a manifestation of His love, His grace, His mercy. If ye would find mercy with God, be merciful to others. If ye would have love with God, love thy fellow man. For as He is love, the earth thereof in light, He gave the new commandment, "Love one another." [See Genesis 1:3, 1:26, and I John 1:5.]

As to the appearances in the earth, these have been few. Not all of these would be given, only those that are a part of the consciousness in the present experience, those controlling or directing that which may be used or rejected in the present consciousness of the entity.

As indicated, be warned regarding fear, its sources and as to how to eliminate same.

Before this the entity was in the land of the present nativity during the early settlings in the "city of brotherly love."

Hence the entity in its inner consciousness in the present is a Quaker, feeling that what is to happen, will happen. What does happen is by the will, then, of that **ye create in thine own consciousness, according to that power ye accredit to that which works within thee.**

The entity was then a teacher, a founder of principles, especially as related to harmonious colors in relationships to individuals.

Hence in the entity's activities, it will find that all of its agreements and activities must be made in the winter months, not in the summer for those have become parts of the entity's consciousness.

Thus the needs for the entity analyzing self, and its abilities may bring to the experience in this present sojourn peace, harmony, as well as material success . . .

5459-3   M.54   6/22/28

Q. How can I overcome the fears that beset me, especially about myself and my wife?

A. *Fear is the root of most of the ills of mankind, whether of self, or of what others think of self, or what self will appear to others.* To overcome fear is to fill the mental, spiritual being, with that which wholly casts out fear; that is, as the love that is manifest in the world through Him who gave Himself the ransom for many. Such love, such faith, such understanding, casts out fear. **Be ye not fearful; for that thou sowest, that thou must reap. Be more mindful of that sown!**

5470-1   F. Adult   9/9/31

Yes, we have the body and those conditions as surround the body. In the physical forces we find the body very good in most respects. There needs be that the mental *body* understand or experience that awakening within, that the body experience the knowledge and an understanding of the relationships between the mental, the physical, and the spiritual body.

In physical forces, or *through* those channels, there have been builded fears, disappointments, and such relations, bringing to the body those ills incident to such conditions. This, in its final analysis, is the lack of faith, hope, and the inability of the body to do *with* pleasure those things it finds hard to do. Hence there is too great a tendency for self-aggrandizement. This must eventually bring its own reward, as would those elements that awaken the spiritual and mental forces of the body, in the final analysis, bring to the physical body *their* own results, from the use of, the applying of, its tenets (those spiritual truths) in the activities of the body itself . . .

Q. What can body do to take away fear of parents' sicknesses?
A. This may only be taken away by *losing* it in *His* power, *His* might, through *spiritual* and *mental* concentration upon the self being a channel of the Creator as thine *own* parents were to *thee*, may you in thine weakness be made strong in, and through *His* might bear those things necessary for that desired.

5563-1   F. Adult   4/24/30

Put self rather, then, in the hands, in the mind, of the *Divine* from within, and not attempting, not *trying* to be good, to be kind, to be thoughtful—but just *be*, and *consecrate* self to the service of others. This peace, this quietness that will come within self from such, will find a ready answer in the mind, in the heart, in the life, in the expression of those—every one— whom the body contacts. *This* is *living* consecration, and not attempting to be moral for moral's sake; not attempting to be good that good may come, but be good that there may be that peace, that understanding, that only comes from putting self in the hands of the Divine. Study, then, portions—*any* portion — of the words of Him that gave that, "That ye ask in my name, *believing*, that shall ye have within yourself." Do not, then, in asking—make conditions—but surrender self unconditionally into the hands of the Divine from within, and that from within shall answer—even as was said, "My spirit beareth witness with your spirit that ye are called the sons, the daughters, of the *living* God," for in Him only is that peace, and the blessings of those whom the body *contacts* will bring the greater joy, the greater happiness. Happiness, then, is not a thing set apart from self, but the conditions with which one approaches that in hand to be *done*! for when one considers that the position of self is hard to bear, is not as is desired, the desire of the heart often maketh one *afraid*—unless that desire is ever in the attitude of *"Use me, O God, as I am,"* for the I AM is ready, willing, to make *my* will *one* with *Thy will*—"Though He slay me, though He bruise me in mine own selfish or unseen ways; yet will I trust Him day by day," and He will *not* forsake thee; neither will He allow thee to be afraid; for He will raise thee up, and He understands all the hardships, the *little* things, the separations, the variations in the surroundings—but *trust* Him!

In this manner may the body, the mental body, the physical body, allow the spirit of truth, peace, joy, understanding, come in and make for self, for those dependent upon self, mentally and physically, whole and strong—and able and capable of meeting every issue of *every* day.

1645-1   F.54   7/22//38

But because of influences from without, or the sensory forces, or the mental reactions that the body makes to circumstances or conditions about it, *fear* has been allowed to enter into the activities of the physical forces. And so oft has the body been told that the disturbance was this or that; and owing to lack of proper eliminations through the alimentary canal and improper influences from other portions of elimination, poisons have been

left until there is fear-poison as well as functional conditions in
the bodily forces themselves.

These all as we find may be materially aided and near to normal conditions result. It will require patience, persistence, faith;
and application *consistently*.

Live and think in constructive ways, *first*!

In the functioning of the organs themselves, **as indicated, we
find that all of the organs of the sensory system are involved;
the hearing, the sight, the taste, the smell — *all* are disturbed at
times.** Unusual odors may occur for the body when they do not
exist to others. An unusual fear or feeling of the presence of this
or that may occur, without the apprehension or understanding of
same from others. The body is disturbed by the hearing of noises,
and the lack of hearing at all other times. The vision is gradually
becoming impaired, physically; as well as the taste.

2056-2   M.38   10/20/27

Q. Give the body any other advice that would be in keeping for
the best development for this body.

A. **Keep thine face toward the light, and the shadows will not
bring fright for fear is the beginning of all undoing. Keep the
heart singing,** and the Lord will raise thee up to *magnify* His
promises to men through service to thine fellow man, for he that
lends to the Lord lays up a store in that realm where thieves do
not break through nor steal. Keep thine ways open, above censure, and *never* censure self.

2205-2   F.37   8/10/40

In analyzing the mental and spiritual attitude of this entity, first
it is well to consider also that which is materially manifested in
the physical body.

**Each entity, each individual, finds that it has a body, a mind,
a soul; each with its attributes, its desires, its hopes, its fears.**

Here we find an entity, an individual, allowing confusions to
arise in such manners because of disappointments and fears —

disappointments in self, and fears as to the attitudes of others.

These are bringing into material manifestation detrimental influences upon the physical being of the entity.

2502-1   F.42   2/26/30

One that is at times easily worried at material things. One that at times worries as respecting the application others make of their abilities. **In the matter of worry, this—in its last analysis—is that of fear. Fear is an enemy to the mental development of an entity, changing or wavering the abilities of an entity in many directions . . .**

In the relationships, the entity finds those conditions often that appear to be contrariwise to that of the desires in self. Long and often has the entity sought for the key to what those presentations are, as are felt innate—and the expressions as are seen from the outside, and how they may be correlated. These often take on those positions where they become as torments, in a manner, to the entity, and there will be seen—from the experiences—*why*, and the application of the will may be the only answer to those questions as often beset the entity; for each and every one, every entity, every individual, every soul—class it or term it as one may, they *mean* the same thing, are to others a difference or a differentiation only according to that classification made within their inner selves—must be able to *satisfy* or *content*, at least, self in its ideal; for there the *ideal* is constantly changed—true, that where the treasure is there is the heart, and the working principle of an individual or entity. **Find that, that is the answer ever for self, as to *an* ideal to be worked toward, to be used at all times, to be leaned upon in adversity and in criticism, in successes, in failures, in pleasures, in hardships, in adversity and in those conditions that are as entanglements of the mental or physical being.** There must be ever the *one* answer, that there *is* the relation between the Maker and that made. There *is* the care *of* the Maker for that created. There is the duty of the created *to* the Creator. There *is* the love for the Creator of that created. There is that of the honor due the Creator *by* that created. The will of the

one must become the will of the other, and *in* that may be found
the answer to *all* questions as disturb; for doth not the Father
take care of all? Then why *worry*? Why be afraid? For "He that
is on the Lord's side, *who* may be against them?" Being one that
trusteth, know in whom thou hast believed, and know that He is
able to keep that committed unto Him against *any* day, *any* time,
any circumstance, *any* condition.

2976-1   M.50   4/20/43

In giving an interpretation of disturbances in the physical forces
of this body, to be the more beneficial to the body it would be
well to consider disturbances with the attitude of the mind of the
individual entity.

**To be sure, there are pathological disturbances here. There
are also psychological reactions.**

When there were the greater distresses, much of that which
arose at the time was of a psychological nature—or the result
of fear. Not merely, in this instance, fear of the results of the
physical effects in the body, but the fear of the results of such a
change for self, as well as the physical fear of those in many ways
associated with the entity's activities.

Thus, in considering how there may be the greater benefits
than are gradually being builded in resistances built up in the
body, we find that the results of attitudes upon pathological
conditions, as well as the effects of radiation, the effects of water,
the effects of air and of fire, will have much to do with the varied
conditions that exist.

Through a general strain that has been produced, and the
result of stresses produced in the physical appetite, and the manner in which and of which there is the supplying to the body of
physical needs—as a result of this fear—a plethoric condition is
produced in the colon of the body.

3650-1   M.66   2/2/44

As we find, there are conditions of which the body should take cognizance. Yet if there is too great a stress, or if there is held in the mental self a fear, there will come those conditions that are spoken of by the Psalmist "That which I feared has come upon me."

Then, apply in nature that which will meet the needs for eliminating any infection that may have been carried in the circulation from those disturbances which have existed. This will in the physical self eliminate the sources, if the fear is eliminated from the mental self that blocks such activity in the living organism in the body.

3658-1   F.40   2/16/44

Q. What is causing the intense pain in the upper back?
A. General nerve reactions to the body—fear.

4082-1   F.52   4/12/44

Q. How did the entity's inferiority complex originate?
A. For the fear or dislike of men. You cannot be one who took the vows and kept them and then lightly turn around and try to gratify the appetites of those who are not easily satisfied.

4610-1   F. Adult   12/18/22

Now, these are the physical conditions as we find them in this body: Through the blood supplying force we find the blood has a tendency toward being overcharged with those elements thrown into the circulation by **fear and produces in the system rather a debilitated condition over the whole body without making a specific organic condition . . .**

4790-1   M. Adult   11/2/23

In the nerve forces there is rather that element of fear and of strained nerve centers than of the nerve system itself, in itself being defective, the body in times back has been in such condi-

tion that the nerve supply of the system was the stronger force within the body. Now fear through the centers, especially in posterior centers of the solar plexus nerve system or branches.

In the organs of the body, we find these conditions: In the brain force, body very good, with the exception of the fear as forms from the centers and gives hallucinations in a form to the cell forces that govern certain portions of the body. Organs of the sensory system, defective in their functioning rather than organic conditions of organs themselves, save that as goes with the condition of the body. In the throat, larynx, bronchials and lungs, we find with the temperature produced in blood by the system attempting to meet the needs of the body, we find these respond spasmodic to the condition. Hence the shortness of breath, the dryness to throat and organs of same, and at times the complaint of secretions troubling these portions of body. Heart overactive at the present time—we find pulsation 95, respiration 32, temperature 98.4

In the digestive forces, we find with the lower portion of the stomach where lacerations have been produced by strangulation of the tissue in these portions of the body—this is where the forces needed by blood supply meet the needs of the condition in the system direct. At present we only have the lacerated condition. These may become other forms of organic conditions, as is signified by the character of the excretions from the system. In this center, too, we find the nerve system overtaxed and the body assimilating fear rather than stimulus of the nature to give relief to the body. That center, the pneumogastric, you see. Duodenum shows the lack of forces assimilated properly. Hence the bacilli created gives to the forces of the lacteal fluids that cause distress through the upper portion of the intestinal tract. Hence, in places or patches [Peyer's patches?] of the intestinal tract itself becoming under this influence, stuff off [slough off?] or show how that the mucus or the inner coating is being attacked by these conditions as created in the pyloric end of the stomach proper. Liver, engorged, and spasmodic in its action of excretory and secretive functioning. Kidneys overcharged, causing the dull, heavy feeling to the abdomen, hips and lower portion of the body.

3474-1   F.22   12/3/43

Q. How can I overcome the social fear which causes me to shun leadership?
A. This is well for the entity, and this ye overcame in the experience before this. Keep it as it is. Don't be a social climber. Don't depend upon social activities. Be a home builder, and the builder of a home.

3509-1   M.29   12/14/43

Q. Career as a pianist was brought to an end through my extreme nervousness and lack of confidence, and other talents have suffered because of an overpowering fear. What am I to do?
A. No doubt overpowering fear. Right about face! Know it is within thee! Defying this has brought the fear, has brought the anxieties. **Turn about, and pray a little oftener. Do this several weeks, yes—let a whole moon pass, or a period of a moon—28 days—and never fail to pray at two o'clock in the morning. Rise and pray—facing east! Ye will be surprised at how much peace and harmony will come into thy soul.** This doesn't mean being goody-goody—it means being good for something, but let it be creative and not that which will eventually turn and rend thee.

5108-1   F.30   5/15/44

Q. How may I overcome the fear I have of falling down steps?
A. Know, as He has given, that He will give His angels charge concerning thee and will bear thee up. **Let that faith, that trust, which has sustained thee in the present, keep thee from fear of any kind.** Not that precautions are not to be taken, for that's what railings are built for! Hold to them, but don't trust them. Trust in the Lord who giveth man judgment and the abilities to those to prepare such!

5226-1   F.58   5/26/44

Q. How can I overcome fear of advancing old age and being alone?

A. **By going out and doing something for somebody else; that is, those not able to do for themselves, making others happy, forgetting self entirely.** These are as material manifestations but in helping someone else you'll get rid of your feelings.

5629-1   F.61   5/11/29

Q. Why have I such fear of noises?

A. The improper coordination between the cerebrospinal and sympathetic system, against these conditions existent in the nerves themselves. Improper reaction of vibratory forces. Hence those conditions as are given for the changes to be exercised by both the action of the Radio-Active Appliance (which is to produce proper coordination in the body) and the active force in that of the Radium Appliance (which acts with the blood and the nerve system, in its exchange of forces as are created by the body for the vibrations through nerve and blood supply, and their relationship one to another).

Forgiveness
792-1   1/15/35

In the application then to the material life, know: **As ye sow, so shall ye reap. With what measure ye mete, it shall be measured to you again.** It is read, "Father, glorify Thou me that I may be glorified before those Thou hast given me, that *they* may be glorified in me."

As ye then forgive those who trespass, who speak evil, who are ungentle, who are unkind, so may the Father forgive thee when *thou* art wayward, when thou art headstrong and seek His face.

These are the laws. These are unchangeable. For He hath

made thee a little lower than the angels, yet at no time hath He said to the angel, "Sit thou on my right side."

Then, if thou wouldst know what may be the understanding heart, just be kind, just be patient, just be lovely, just be friendly to thy fellow man. *Forgive* those that speak lightly or unkindly, or who even in premeditated manner do thee evil. For if ye forgive not these, how can thy heavenly Father forgive thee?

793-2   F.53   8/27/36

When anger hath beset thee, hast thou stopped and considered what the fruit of rash words would bring? Hast thou not said, "Yes, I forgive but I cannot forget. Yes, I will not remember but don't remind me of what you did."

How hath it been given? If ye would be forgiven, ye must forgive. If ye would know love, ye must be lovely. If ye would have *life, give* it! What is life? *God!*—in action with thy fellow man!

Love
38-1   F.5   6/23/28

In the control, one that may be reasoned with, but rarely commanded without reason given for such command.

One that may be *loved* into doing or becoming that as would guide the entity, and rarely forced—either by circumstance or by conditions—to adhere to principle or to percept without that love being shown or manifested in the directing.

One that with Jupiter and Uranus influence, will be found to be exceptional in abilities toward those arts, or elements of life that go to make up the characteristics of the developing personality as manifested in the present experience. Here (as a side note) may be given, there is manifested in this entity that which may perfectly illustrate that difference between personality and individuality, as the individual with urge as must be directed.

Those of exceptional abilities with Uranian influence may be *well* said also to mean exceptional abilities to err, or to be led astray in the direction not best for self or self's development.

One with the ability to be exceptional as a musician. One that may use this same ability to entice, overpower, to subdue, to subjugate others *to* the power, unless guided, directed, and *loved into* the correct idea of the use of power in any and all directions . . .

. . . In the one before this we find in the land now known as Persia. The entity then among those of the school that were destroyed by the invaders from the now Arabian and Egyptian country. The entity was one that was loved by the king's daughter, and one that gave self rather than see that friend fall into the hands of the invaders; yet prevented it not. Gaining, then, in this experience—and true may it be said of this entity, a love child. In the name Ibseor. In the urge as seen from this experience, again good and bad. That of the urge to be slow in making friendships, yet when once made the entity gives *all* in the defense or succor of same.

262-44   4/30/33

The first lesson that each must learn: Love is the giving out of that within self.

Then, where slights, slurs, or even suspicions, have been allowed to enter in as respecting the fellow man, there cannot be all of what love should be, should mean, in the experience of such an one.

For, "He so loved the world as to give His own son." And it has been asked of everyone, "Love me, keep my commandments, that I may abide in thee even as I abide in the Father."

All believe, yes; all know, yes; all understand that those things that hinder each and every soul are only self-centeredness, selfishness in self, that prevent even the dawn of that concept of what love means in their experience.

All see in various activities in the earth that of maternal love, that of love in friendship, that of love for an ideal, for self, for the varied experiences that are seen in everyone's experience.

Yet, to know the whole truth that makes one free indeed; that love that prevents slurs, slights, unkind remarks, falterings here, disappointments there—in things, in people, in

conditions; to not shake faith, the foundation of manifesting in the material experience; few have found this.

1472-13   F.61   5/3/41

Q. Why is my love and concern for my grandson,[...]so much greater than it is for my granddaughter,[...]?
A. In those associations with each of these through the Palestine experience, there were those periods in which there was the ability of the one to be self-sufficient—which brings an indifference; while the seeking for counsel, for help, or for instruction in the other, naturally brings the greater feeling of response. For, it is a universal and a divine law that like begets like. So, in the present experience, while there is loving—yet in the one it might be truly called loving indifference, while in the other it is love that is truly a creative, growing experience in the activities of each.

1579-1   G.34   4/27/38

While each soul, each associate, each acquaintance *is* an obligation, a duty—all of these must cooperate, coordinate. As the body itself in its welfare, mentally or physically, unless it cooperates, coordinates each portion with the other, there is not the well-rounded, the well-balanced individual nor the better and best reactions from same.

There is the physical body, there is the mental body, there is the spiritual body. They are one. They each have their attributes. They each have their weaknesses. They each have their associations. Yet they must be all coordinated.

The spirit is the life. Then each phase of the experience of the entity must be of the spiritual import in its very nature, if it is to live, to be the fulfilling of its purpose—to bring peace and harmony, for which purpose it *is* in existence! It must be constructive in the very nature and the very desires, without thought of self being the one glorified in or by same! Rather the *glory* is to the influence or force that *prompts* same!

As is the experience in the entity: If even filial or marital or soul love seeks the exalting of self, then it is not fulfilling its purpose from the spiritual import. God is love! The influence or force that motivates the life of each soul is love! But it may be love of self, of fame, of fortune, of glory, of beauty, or of self-indulgence, self-aggrandizement, or the satisfaction to the ego!

1616-1   F.44   6/14/38

The entity has loved well materially; not always wisely. For being so intuitive, so loving as to be taken advantage of, the results have not been in keeping with the intent. Hence it has been given to such, "Be ye wise as serpents but harmless as doves," speaking evil of none; finding whereunto there is rather the *cooperative* point of contact with each phase of human experience and human endeavor, knowing and realizing that no power exists save as is allowable by the Father.

1632-3   F.38   8/9/38

As in Venus — the love of the beautiful; the appreciation of efforts on the part of others; the inclinations for social activities, as related to the expressions of love — of the manifestations. **And while the entity will find that all love is lawful, of every nature, not** *all* **is** *expedient* **unto good works.**

1821-1   M.54   2/14/39

Love, in its greatest aspect, does not *possess!* **It** *is!* **It is not then possessive, to be real . . .**
Q. Should I go on in the friendship for a certain family in Boston, with whom I spend much time, and can I help them further to find or know important truths or to find themselves?
A. This is very good — just so it does not become possessive.

1828-1   F.20   2/21/39

For, as has been indicated so oft, ye *are* what ye are because of how ye have applied thy opportunities in filling those purposes for which the Giver of all good and perfect gifts brought thee into awareness, even in the physical *and* mental and spiritual realms.

Then it behooves each entity to so live as to never have questionings within self as to whether or not that which is desired is for the best; but have *proofs* of same! **Never be in that attitude of censuring; leaving off entirely those inclinations to censure others.**

For, remember, truth and goodness need no justification, only *glorification* to God in the *manner* of dealings with thy fellow man.

Show patience, show mercy, as ye would have these shown to thee! Show brotherly kindness—and above all *love*; **not possessive, but** *love***—as ye** *would* **depict same, in thy abilities to indicate same upon activities of individuals or things or conditions.**

2011-1   F.37   9/23/39

From the very nature and the liking of change, oft the entity has been called fickle or insecure; and yet capable of and desiring the thrill of a great love experience in the material life.

Let it be based, too, upon spiritual concepts if you would know or experience or have this great love to be a reality.

2174-2   F.50   1/29/41

How well ye will meet the problems as they are presented depends upon how well ye have mastered, and do master, the problems before thee from day to day.

In Him, the Christ, as manifested in Jesus, ye find this—the first, the greatest commandment—Thou shalt love the Lord thy God (that as manifested in self *as* life itself), and thy neighbor as thyself."

That which brings these both in awareness is that so well and yet so badly named *love*. God is love. An individual entity, each soul, each entity, each body, finds the need of expressing that called love in the material experience; from its first awareness until its last call through God's other door—the need of love, expressed, manifested, by self and from others.

As ye sow, so shall ye reap—this again becomes the foundation of what self, as well as others may expect. If ye would have friends, show thyself friendly; if ye would have love, love ye one another. These are unchangeable. They do not alter. Man alters them only in the application—as to whether it is to satisfy the ego or the animal, or the flesh, or the mind.

These expressions, then, to self, as is experienced in motherhood, give the greatest glory manifested in the earth.

Thus may ye indeed know such, as **ye mete it out to others.**

2364-1   F.27   9/2/31

With the ideals as come through those of Venus, a *lovable* disposition; one easily making friends, yet—with all—a tendency that must be warred against, of the inclination of selfish interests; not that these may not be warred against, nor that self may not apply itself in a way and manner—but as to the ideal as is set before self, this will make for that as will be builded as a life that must be gratified in those things that partake of earth, or whether those that partake of the spiritual life, those that partake of the mental life. **Hence the ideals that the entity sets before self, the goals the entity expects and attempts to attain, will make for those conditions as will bring that that makes for contentment and peace, or whether they bring those conditions that with use wear away.** Oft has it been said, and *well* were it that all consider friendships and loves that are builded on peace *grow*, while those things that partake of earth become weather-worn, and with age unfit, unuseful; yet those that partake of those things that bespeak of the abilities that come with love *in* its higher sense *build*, grow more beautiful as time, age, comes on. In this, then, will the entity do well, that those things that become as the thoughtful portions of its activities, in the little things that the body busies itself with, that they partake more and more of that not *always* as *sacrifices*; for, as has oft been said, no longer does the Higher

Force, or God, call for sacrifice; rather that ye love on another, even with that love as was shown in the gift of the *Holy* One, that we through Him might have access *to* the Father, *to* the throne of mercy and of grace! In giving, living, *being*—then—that as draws nearer to these characterizations in activities in and out before men, may *all*—even as this entity—find that peace, that contentment, that comes with knowing that the whole armor is put on, having the feet shod with a joyous message, having on the helmet of light, with hands ever ready to lend a *helping* hand to *everyone*, in *every* manner. In *this* characterization of an ideal may the entity meet and make for those developments *in* the present, that are characterized in those influences *in* Neptune; not as mysteries not understood, but rather as being, living, doing, those things *through* those channels that *brings* the understanding of the glorious love of Him, shed in a world of sin!

3573-1   F.28   12/28/43

In interpreting the records here, then, we find Mars, Venus, Jupiter and Uranus as part of the experience.

Mars—anger, activity. **The entity will ever be busy, with its hands, with its mind. And these need, then, more direction not in material things but in spiritual.**

In Venus we find that the entity passes through those experiences of beauty, art; yet these oft take the turns for material expressions—and these the entity tends to embrace. Let them rather be lost in His purposes. Let love be without dissimulation, and not so much centralized in individuals or personalities, nor in self. Love is universal, as God. Crystallized it is beautiful, but minimized in selfishness or spread abroad in the aggrandizement of self becomes those stumbling blocks over which many tumble into restlessness for gratification, for activities to satisfy self.

3744-5   2/14/24

Q. What is the law of love?
A. **Giving**. As is given in this injunction, "Love thy neighbor as

thyself." As is given in the in the injunction, "Love the Lord thy God with all thine heart, thine soul and thine body." In this, as in many, we see upon the physical or earth or material plane the manifestations of that law, without the law itself. With any condition we find as this, which is the manifestation of the opposite from law of love. The gift, the giving, with hope of reward or pay is direct opposition of the law of love. Remember—there is no greater than the injunction, "God so loved His creation, or the world, as to give His only begotten Son, for their redemption." Through that love, as man makes it manifest in his own heart and life, does it reach that law, and in compliance of *a* Law, the law becomes a part of the individual. *That is the law of love.* **Giving in action, without the force felt, expressed, manifested, shown, desired, or reward for that given. Not that the law of love does away with other laws, but makes** *the law of recompense, the law of faith, the law of divine, with the law of earth forces,* **if you please, of effect, not defective, but of effect.**

So we have *love* is *law, law is love. God is love. Love is God.* In that we see the law manifested, not the law itself. Unto the individual, as we have given then, that gets the understanding of self, becomes a part of this. As is found, which come in one, so we have manifestations of the one-ness, of the all-ness in love. Now, if we, as individuals, upon the earth plane, have all of the other elementary forces that make to the bettering of life, and have not love we are as nothing—nothing. "Though one may have the gift of prophecy, so as to give great understanding, even of the graces in hope, in charity, in faith, and has not the law of love in their heart, soul, mind and though they give their body to give itself for manifesting even these graces, and has not love—they are nothing." In many, many ways may the manifestations of the law of love be shown, but without the greater love, even as the Father giveth, even as the soul giveth, there is no understanding, and no compliance of the forces that make our later law to this, of effect.

3954-1   F.71   11/5/43

Q. What is meant by learning the law of love? How may I do this?

A. It is that ye make applicable in thy daily experiences. "Love me" is ever the command. "A new commandment I give, that ye love one another even as I have loved you." It is the willingness to sacrifice all of self, even the abilities of self, that others may know the Lord better.

Attitudes and Emotions
Part III
Optimism
137-7   M.26   11/19/24

Q. How can he put his finances in such a condition as to permit him to concentrate to his greatest possibility on his psychic development?

A. **Be not dismayed, for the development in psychic forces must manifest in and through the present conditions, and conditions physical, financial, must of necessity be one and a part of the development.** As is given in this: In whatsoever state one finds (as he has found himself) oneself, make self content; not satisfied, but content, ever working toward that oneness of mind (of body, of will, with the development), or universal, or psychic forces. Do not war against these conditions. **Make of conditions the stepping-stones to the development necessary to meet the daily needs in physical, in mental, in financial.**

137-127   M.31   2/1/6/30

Q. My feeling regarding the financial affairs and all those connected dependent on this financial affair—is my liberal and optimistic viewpoint correct?

A. Correct, so long as they abide in that that brings for that purposefulness as is seen in thine own self; for, as it has been given, there lies within self that *ability*, that *consciousness* of purpose, for the self to become one that may wield a greater influence in the financial affairs of the world than of *any one individual* now *in* the earth's plane. **That's optimism!**

257-183   M.44   5/24/37

Q. What is best plan to keep health and mental attitude good, considering location of home?
A. As has so oft been given, budget the time, the abilities, the facilities. Do not overtax one at the expense of the other.

Keep joyous, keep optimistic; but do not overpower, do not exaggerate self or self's associations to such an extent as to become boring to those who can only think in a few dollars!

462-10   M.51   5/20/36

Q. Was the experience that I have gone through necessary?
A. **Unless the entity, unless the body looks upon the experiences day by day as necessary influences and forces, and uses them as a stepping-stone, soon does life become a pessimistic outlook.** If each and every disappointment, each and every condition that arises, is used as a stepping-stone for better things and looking for it and expecting it, then there will still be continued the optimism. Or the looking for and expecting of. If an individual doesn't expect great things of God, he has a very poor God, hasn't he?

533-14   M.26   5/12/37

In the mental and spiritual, be more constructive and not too passive—or not too positive in unconstructive ways. Not that the attitude is so destructive, but it should not be so active in *unconstructive* ways! **In other words, do not be so pessimistic. Be more optimistic; always.**

540-11   F.35   10/11/38

And keep that attitude which has been a part of the entity's whole mental being, mien and manner. Know that the body creates, or will revive itself. Then keep that attitude of optimism and helpfulness to others, and it makes the environment of then the same for self. **Worry more about somebody else than you do about** yourself, and you'll be a lot better off!

551-13   M.36   5/15/34

Q. How is my mental condition, and how can it be improved?
A. The mental condition is in that state where a great deal of the temperamental and the nervous reactions are allowed by the self dwelling upon immediate surroundings. If the body will train or *make* self, as it were, by sheer will force, to see conditions rather as the whole than as individual case or condition, there will be a much better reaction to the whole mental outlook.

Know that the circumstances or conditions through which the body may pass are or can be used by the body as a stepping-stone for the bettered conditions. For, there should be rather the attitude that, "If I myself keep my mind upon those things that have to deal with the spiritual aspects of a physical life, that find their expression in the reaction of individuals to individuals, then the growth of same is in the attitude I hold to my associations in each activity."

Be rather of the optimistic outlook, for there you may find that the growth of self is in keeping with how that expenditure of self is made in such directions.

Not to that of extravagance in *any* thought or activity; but that which is in keeping with those things that have oft been given; if ye would have friends, make self friendly with all thou mayest meet in *every walk* of life.

If thou wouldst have shown forth to thee that of brotherly love, then show same to thy friend, thy neighbor, thine enemy, thine stranger, that ye meet day by day.

Such will make for growth, for the attraction of the proper relationships in the experiences and affairs of *any* individual.

1700-1   M.11   10/4/38

Too easily may the entity become pessimistic; and he will find sooner or later that the optimist finds greater happiness, much greater joy in living.

1804-1   M.52   1/28/39

One that will find music as an outlet for self in a great many ways and manners.

And whenever there are the periods of depression, or the feeling low or forsaken, play music; especially stringed instruments of every nature. These will enable the entity to span that gulf as between pessimism and optimism.

Keep optimistic as much as possible. Know that as ye give out ye receive, and that alone as ye have given away do ye possess.

2573-1   M.33   8/12/41

The entity has two distinct natures, and at times appears to be very optimistic and at others very pessimistic. This at times causes some disturbance in the minds of those with whom the entity is associated. Apparently, to some, the entity is inconsistent.

The virtue of consistency should be nourished, or the lack of it corrected. For as the entity journeys through life he should minimize the faults and magnify the virtues; not only in self and self's relationships to things to conditions and to individuals, but also minimize the faults and magnify the virtues to the associates.

Thus the halfway mark, or the being temperate in the pessimism and the optimism would be a lesson for the entity to attain.

3420-1   F.57   12/17/43

And unless each soul entity (and this entity especially) makes the world better, that corner or place of the world a little better, a little bit more hopeful, a little bit more patient, showing a little more of brotherly love, a little more of kindness, a little more of long-suffering—by the very words and deeds of the entity, the life is a failure; especially so far as growth is concerned. **Though you gain the whole world, how little ye must think of thyself if ye lose the purpose for which the soul entered this particular sojourn!**

Think not more highly of thyself that ye ought to think, yet no one will think more of you than you do of yourself; not in egotism, but in the desire to be of a help. **For who is the greatest? He that is the servant of all, he that contributes that which makes each soul glad to be alive, glad to have the opportunity to contribute something to the welfare of his brother. These are thy virtues or thy faults, dependent upon how ye use them.**

The entity then naturally should ever be an optimist, not a pessimist.

Pessimism
3440-2   M.36   12/20/43

The entity oft tends to become a bit pessimistic and to blame someone else. This is not well. For every tub, yes every cup, must sit upon its own bottom, its own legs. For since the giving of the Son of God Himself that man might be reconciled to God, no man pays for the sins of others. It is all in self—in self. For He came to save all.

3528-1   M.36   12/20/43

The entity becomes very sensitive at times, and at such times becomes aggravated, flies off the handle as it were, says things it doesn't mean, but is so sincere that if it has spoken a word it will stick to it though it hurts all the while. Hardheaded, pessimistic. These are the faults. Correct these in thy associations. First have a reason for correcting them, not merely that ye may be well-spoken of, not merely that ye may get along with people, but because it is right! For remember, every virtue has its own reward—in the application of that virtue in the experience with others . . .

And as ye find in thyself, it is only thyself from which ye are to be saved—hardheadedness and your pessimism! . . .

Remember, if ye would gain from such ye must also contribute to same. For ye may gain only so much as ye contribute to any society, organization or group, whatever it may be. For each individual is made in the image of creation, and unless ye are a creator in such ye are taking from same. If ye are taking from same, it lessens and lessens the abilities in every phase of the experience to be a permanent success. For the attitude of "Gimmie—Gimmie" and never a giver leads only to a miserable failure in the long run. If you would have life you must give life. If you would have friends you must be friendly. If you would have love you must yourself be lovely. And in so doing ye will discard selfishness and pessimism—that is so much a part of thyself...

Learn by mental as well as material experience. Do not be such a pessimist nor such a materialist.

5264-1   F.40   6/14/44

As we find, there are many complimentary experiences latent and manifested in the urges of this body, and there are those which at times cause a great deal of anxiety to the body.

For as we find, while very optimistic as to life, as to its experiences, as to the hopes, as to the joys, as to the desires, at times apparently without a cause, pessimism takes hold, and without the desire on the part of the entity, everything apparently seems useless.

These, then are both good and bad, for the entity finds at times, when even it is with its loved ones and those for whom it cares the most, suddenly it will appear as being alone or lonesome and have the desire for changes, though the body may be quiet, may be content. Not that the body seeks extraordinary social experiences, but these seem at times futile and again so very necessary.

Hence, we find a condition to be reckoned with in the experience of the entity: to learn, to gain, to acquire, to be truly content in that which the entity sets as its highest ideal in spiritual, in mental, in material things. This done, we may have a great deal more harmonious experiences in this sojourn in the earth.

5302-1   M.35   6/28/44

In giving the interpretations of the records, there is much to choose from and while that which may be given here may appear as condemning, this takes not from the latent and the manifested abilities which are manifested in this entity; yet there are those tendencies for this entity to see only the dark side of any experiences. The entity is pessimistic as to the outcome of any venture. **These should be rather replaced with the mind building to see the lessons in pointed stories, or in those told more in the manner of dispensation of periods, or when changes are wrought in the experience.**

Thus, as we find, there may be made those associations, those connections wherein the entity will read a great many funny papers, or the whole attention of the mind should be turned to Creative Forces which would bring about the opportunities for the possibilities which are latent and manifest in the experiences of this entity.

These experiences are too oft allowed to be pushed aside or be considered, "Well, that's what he thinks."

Think then, for self; know God is not mocked and whatsoever a man soweth, that must he reap. If ye feel sorry for self, is there any help? **If ye would be a man, be manly! If ye would have friends, act friendly! If ye would have love, manifest same in thy relationships with others! and these bring fruits which may be the greater contributing factors in the entity finding itself.**

Righteousness
1770-2   F.49   12/29/38

As the entity has advanced and does advance in its concept of or awareness of the creative influences within its experience, then those things that have been and are as a part of the mental self are to be met or overcome or conquered, or used; and there is the understanding of how to use, then, as it were, the tools of righteousness or of salvation in a material plane.

These oft become very delicate in their nature (if words were to be used to express their influence or motivating power within the experience of an entity), yet they *are* the tools of righteousness.

3621-1   F.8   1/7/44

In analyzing the urges latent and manifested, we would magnify the virtues and minimize the faults. This, too, should be that lesson of greater importance in the developing mind of this entity; else the entity—as may be indicated from the character of the experiences—may become self-centered, and this would be to the detriment of the greater development of this entity. Magnify the virtues of all, as ye would have thy God, thy Maker, magnify thy trying, thy attempts to be holy—not righteous; so few can ever attain that—none in the material world—[but] they can try. **All can be holy; that is, dedicating body, mind and purpose. That is being holy!**

Then, the try may be counted to thee as righteousness. For righteousness is of God.

5749-13   3/12/41

Then, let all so examine their hearts and minds as to put away doubt and fear; **putting away hate and malice, jealousy and those things that cause man to err. Replace these with the desire to help, with hope, with the willingness to divide self and self's surroundings with those who are less fortunate; putting on the whole armor of God**—in righteousness.

Magnify in the daily life the fruit of the spirit of truth, that all may take hold and make for that activity in their lives; knowing that as ye do it unto the least of thy brethren ye do it to thy Maker.

There are hundreds of other discussions of Attitudes and Emotions in the Cayce trilogy, but I think this gives you a good beginning discussion to make decisions for your future! As you digest this multidimensional view of attitudinal/emotional problems, be aware that in general, all of them are the result of your genetic, familial, environmental conditioning. **You are responsible not only for your unhealthy reactions and beliefs but also for optimizing them!** In a later chapter I will also give you some suggested mental exercises.

6

Archetypes of
the Elements

If we are aware of the subtle nature of everything, we begin to appreciate the archetypal, mythic, symbolic nature so abundant in nature itself. The inherent pervasiveness of nature as part of life force is seen in the widespread use of fire, air, earth, and water in folk medicine. And of course, the Chinese also included metal. Having received from guides the 5 Sacred Rings: Fire, Air, Water, Earth, and Crystal, I recently began to look at their archetypal meanings.

Fire

The discovery of fire itself is responsible for one of the great archetypal transformations of civilization. For many foods, cooking enhances nutrient availability and assists in decreasing putrefaction. And of course it provides warmth in cold weather. Fire, above all, represents energy, including life energy and electricity. Fire chemicals are cortisone, adrenalin, and dehydroepiandrosterone, DHEA. DHEA represents our stress reserves or adrenal reserve. Low DHEA is a sign of adrenal burnout. The fire signs in astrology are Aries and Mars, the God of War; Leo and the Sun; and Sagittarius, associated with good and noble and a higher purpose, each associated with concepts of great energy. Fire is the wizard, creator, light, heat, goodness, and positive energy.

Diseases of fire are:
- Depression—lack of fire
- Rheumatoid arthritis and inflammatory diseases—too much fire which is imbalanced
- Hypertension—too much fire
- Migraine—imbalanced fire
- Diabetic neuropathy—loss of fire
- Pain—too much or too little fire

Air

Air is the breath of life, universal power, purity. In fact, the brain dies if it does not receive fresh air/oxygen within three minutes. Air represents the archetypal hero. Inspiration, imagination, and intuition are crucial aspects of air energy. Logic, freedom, language, and flight are air energies. Air signs are Aquarius, the butterfly chasing the rainbow, associated with Uranus, associated with rebirth, experimentation, and sometimes hubris; Gemini, the twin who has difficulty sometimes deciding on the flow of life and associated with Mercury, the God of Travel; and Libra, the disciple of right and wrong, associated with Venus, the Goddess of love.

Diseases of air:
- Hearing problems
- Tinnitus, deafness
- Lung diseases, asthma, COPD, emphysema, etc.
- Autism, coupled with earth
- ADHD, coupled with earth
- Down's Syndrome, coupled with earth
- Fainting
- The psyche

Water

Water is second only to air in essentials for life, the most primal of all archetypes. It is fluid, changeable, associated with emotions and especially with heart and kidneys, with the unconscious mind, with cleansing and rebirth, and with spirit, the source of life. It is associated with fertility, circulation, and purity. The water signs are Pisces, the fish swimming in both directions and with Neptune, the God of the oceans and of water; Cancer (I prefer to call it the moon child), associated with home and nurturing, caring, associated with the Divine Mother and the moon, the hidden emotions; and Scorpio, the secretive, sexual, the manipulating and the most intelligent and associated with Pluto, God of the Underworld.

Diseases of water:
- Congestion and congestive heart failure
- Kidney failure
- Diabetes insipidus
- Swelling
- Obesity
- Great emotions, positive and negative

Earth

Above all earth is being grounded, real, productive, the Earth Mother, protector, mediator, peacemaker, harmony, a balance of yin and yang. Earth signs are Taurus, the mythical Ferdinand the Bull, warm, kind, and supportive associated with Venus, the Goddess of Love; Virgo, the most organized and another Earth Mother, Aphrodite, and associated with Mercury, God of speed, travel, music; and Capricorn the most capricious, loyal, trustworthy, prudent, organized and associated with Saturn, Ruler of the world, master, both a tyrant and wise old man.

Earth diseases:
- Chronic fatigue
- Fibromyalgia
- Paralysis

- Most neurologic diseases, ALS, Parkinsonism, etc.
- Stroke
- Cancer
- Many immune diseases
- Seduction
- Kidney and liver diseases

Crystal

The symbol of Higher Consciousness. The Mystic, Professor, Student. Crystals receive, store, and transmit energy. Crystalline energy is for regeneration and overall energy balancing
.

Diseases of Crystal energy:
- Degenerative diseases
- Wear and tear problems
- Co-factors with Earth diseases

Supernoetics™—See www.supernoetics.com for more details.

As I said in the beginning, it is impossible to separate body, mind, and soul. One of the best overviews is Dr. Keith Scott-Mumby's Glass Elevator Mind model.

Universal Consciousness—At the top of the elevator is consciousness, which he considers "awareness of awareness." You can "watch" your stream of thoughts, emotions, etc.

Own consciousness is just below consciousness—awareness that we are a "cloud of conscious entities, operating in the same psychic space," almost multiple personalities which can have "coexisting contrary attitudes." We have an illusion that we have a single mind, since the multiple thoughts appear to our mind to come from the same identi-fication! *Ultimate insight here is a true spiritual experience.*

The Self-Complex is below the "cloud consciousness"—thought itself. Essentially, you can change your thoughts by changing the words you use! You can think happy or angry or sad, etc.

Emotions are the physical feelings we experience with our thoughts! Dr. Scott-Mumby discusses this "Ladder of Emotions in Supernoetics™.

Neural Nets are the bio-energetic complexes that essentially integrate the multiple mental-physical reactions which become patterns of thinking/feeling, such as sexual activity and religious beliefs that have been acculturated through years of habitual reactions and to some extent brain-washing.

Animal thinking is the basic will to survive: "eating, safety, and pro-creation." These biological essentials "stand in the way of our spiritual life"—and may indeed shatter it!

7

Restoring Health— Healing

Even with the best of conscientious habits, things happen. We have the potential of genetic predispositions, karmic influences, accidents, and many social as well as environmental influences that can lead to illnesses or diseases not the result of unhealthy habits. And, of course, we also have the possibility of problems that are definitely because we chose healthy habits too late in life! For instance, perhaps we smoked for five years in our early adulthood, drank excessively, did not exercise adequately, etc. All of these predispose us to virtually every conceivable illness. Hypertension, heart disease, diabetes, and cancer are significantly "caused" by those unhealthy habits. And they equally may have genetic or karmic roots. And, of course, chlorinated water and fluoridated water are major toxins that eventually take their toll, as do the not-so-obvious chemicals polluting our food supply. Then there are still dentists doing silver amalgam fillings which pour mercury into our bodies. And don't forget plain old smog! Assuming you have less than ten symptoms on the Symptom Index and that you feel well, there are some periodic evaluations to consider. Many of these are **not** even thought of by the average physician.

Self-Testing

Men
Palpate testicles once a month.
Visually check your skin in a full length mirror once a month.
Check your weight once a month, if your weight is "normal—Body Mass Index 18–24.

Women
Palpate your breasts once a week.
Visually check your skin in a full length mirror once a month.
Check your weight once a month, if your weight is "normal—Body Mass Index 18–24.

By age 20
Blood test for homocysteine
Blood pressure, CBC, and SMAC chemical panel

Age 35, 50, 65
Repeat tests of age 20 plus
Stool test for blood
Coronary calcium score

At age 50 get an ADMA test—Asymmetric Dimethyl Arginine and men have a prostate exam

Adrenal Fatigue or Burnout

Chronic fatigue is one of the best indicators of stress burnout. Laboratory wise, the best test is a free DHEA and I recommend **only** Nichols Lab in Capistrano, California for this. There is a simple home test that you might do to know that you are burned out:

Blood Pressure and Pulse

Lie down and relax for twenty minutes. Take your blood pressure and pulse. Stand up and recheck BP and pulse. Blood pressure should go up 10 or 20 points as should pulse. If BP falls and pulse goes up more than 20 points, you have adrenal fatigue. The best antidote is autogenic training, as discussed much earlier. In addition there are some supplements worth considering:

Ashwagandha, 500 mg

Panax Ginseng, 500 mg

Of course Fire Bliss, magnesium lotion, Youth Formula and natural progesterone also help restore DHEA!!

And, of course, in addition to autogenic training, there are a number of additional insight exercises worth doing:

After ten minutes of autogenic training, sense your overall relationship with your mother. Do you have unfinished business with her? Anger, guilt anxiety, or sadness? Are you willing to forgive her? Are you willing to bless her for giving you life?

On another occasion, after initial AT, sense your relationship with your father. Is there unfinished business—anger, guilt, anxiety, or depression? Are you willing to forgive him? Are you willing to bless him for giving you life?

Continue this practice with all the people in your life with whom you need healing!

Once you have truly come to grips with all the people in your life, you are ready to get in touch with you! Are you willing to forgive and bless yourself? Then, the major exercise is to repeat and believe:

> *I have a body, and I am more than my body.*
> *I have emotions, and I am more than my emotions.*
> *I have a mind, and I am more than my mind.*
> *At my innermost being, I am magnificent, wise and loving.*

Create a symbolic image of the real you, your soul—a magnificent sky-blue five-pointed star beaming down upon you its perfect soul power. Recognize that your body is indeed the temple of your soul!

Once you can do this and MEAN it, you are ready to connect with

God, which you may imagine as a giant white six-pointed star beaming down upon you and the world as a perfect golden-orange light.

Beyond Body, Mind, and Activity

Although there is great concern among many people about vaccines, I do believe that the most basic vaccines are valuable in childhood—DPT, tetanus, polio. I am not at all certain that I can routinely recommend others, and I do **not** recommend flu shots or shingles vaccines. Instead I recommend that all adults routinely take:

- Vitamin D 3, 50,000 units once a week if you weigh 140 or more pounds. If you are between 90 and 135 pounds, take 50,000 units every two weeks.
- Vitamin K 2, 100 micrograms daily.
- A good multivitamin/mineral with 25 mg each of B 1,2,3,6 and trace minerals.
- Omega-3, 1000 mg daily.

When You Need to See a Physician

Conventional medicine shines in acute care. Please do not ignore the following:

- Fainting
- Significant bleeding
- Major injuries
- Pregnancy
- Significant alterations in consciousness
- Major personality changes
- Sudden severe pain
- A sudden fever above 103 degrees
- Inability to empty bladder or to have a bowel movement
- Severe diarrhea/dysentery
- Severe vomiting
- Significant unexplained weight loss

Now take the following self-evaluations:

SPIRITUAL COMPETENCE
On a scale of zero to 4, how adequately competent are you? Maximum score is 60!

0–4 (Maximum)

	0	1	2	3	4
1. I am fully able to take care of myself.					
2. I complete any task I have started.					
3. I understand my problems.					
4. I handle personal challenges/problems well.					
5. I make a positive contribution to the world.					
6. I have a strong sense of purpose in life.					
7. I believe in continuity of life after physical death.					
8. I do quiet introspection daily.					
9. I am open to new insights.					
10. I am non-judgmental but discriminating.					
11. I forgive those who insult me.					
12. I am joyful.					
13. I tolerate people with other beliefs that do not harm me.					
14. I feel at peace.					
15. I believe that the purpose of life is good.					

SPIRITUAL WELL-BEING
On a scale of zero to 4, how adequately competent are you? Maximum score is 60!

0–4 (Maximum)

	0	1	2	3	4
1. Forgiving					
2. Tolerant					
3. Serene/at peace					
4. Compassionate					
5. Charitable					
6. Motivated					
7. Joyous					
8. Certain of a purpose in life					
9. Hopeful for the future					
10. Confident					
11. Courageous					
12. Ability to express needs/desires					
13. Logical					
14. Wise in choices					
15. Unconditionally Loving					

HUMAN POTENTIAL ATTITUDE INVENTORY

As you read each of the following items to yourself, get a sense of whether your emotional response is agreement or disagreement. If you get a strong disagreement, mark 0. If you get a mild agreement, mark 1. If you get a moderate agreement, mark 2. If you get a fairly strong agreement, mark 3. If you get a very strong agreement, mark 4. It sometimes happens that people are in agreement in general and are simultaneously aware of an uneasy feeling that argues, or their brain shows them a single exception. In such a case, it is permissible to answer 1 or 2, which would be preferable to marking 0 if you are really getting a mixed response.

	0-4 (Maximum)
	0 | 1 | 2 | 3 | 4
1. I have forgiven everyone who has wronged me.	| | | | | |
2. I forgive those who unintentionally wrong me.	| | | | | |
3. I forgive those who purposefully wrong me.	| | | | | |
4. When I tell those who have wronged me what they have done, I expect them to apologize or repent.	| | | | | |
5. I have sometimes wronged or harmed others.	| | | | | |
6. I apologize when I wrong others.	| | | | | |
7. I expect others to forgive me when I apologize.	| | | | | |
8. I helped someone else within the last week.	| | | | | |
9. I walked and talked with someone I love during the last week.	| | | | | |
10. I attend church regularly.	| | | | | |
11. I believe that my attitude each day is more important than attending church.	| | | | | |
12. I believe my affliction(s) was/were given to me by God for his honor and glory as part of a divine plan.	| | | | | |
13. I believe God is wrathful and punishes sinners.	| | | | | |

	0	1	2	3	4
14. I have lots of friends and see/visit them often.					
15. I pray regularly for myself and others.					
16. I believe the most important goal of life is service to God or others.					
17. I prayed for someone else yesterday or today.					
18. I often (more than once a week) watch sunset and sunrise with a feeling of reverence.					
19. I read the Bible or inspirational materials at least once a week.					
20. I attend a fun event or listen to good music at least once a week.					
21. I meditate, pray, or think about the beauty of life regularly.					
22. Everyone is born a sinner.					
23. Mankind is basically bad.					
24. I believe hypnosis is the work of the Devil.					
25. I believe everyone has a right to his or her beliefs.					
26. I believe that those who do not share my religious beliefs are sinners and likely to go to Hell.					
27. God does not forgive sinners unless the debts of sins are paid.					
28. If your beliefs are different from mine, you cannot help me.					
29. My spiritual/religious beliefs are: a. strong ____ b. correct or right____					
30. I feel calm and serene most of the time.					
31. When I become frustrated, I pause and calm myself.					
32. I feel compassion for all other human beings.					
33. I go out of my way to help other persons.					
34. I know I can attain my goals.					

	0	1	2	3	4

35. I believe I can accomplish anything to which I apply myself adequately.

36. I will apply myself enough to accomplish my goals.

37. I feel great joy in my life.

38. I can face whatever life offers.

39. I believe I learn from my problems.

40. I willingly or lovingly contribute to help others less fortunate than I.

41. I believe tomorrow will be a better day.

42. I believe in a benevolent God.

43. I believe in life after death.

44. I believe I have a soul that survives death.

45. I believe one dies and goes to Heaven or Hell.

46. I believe in reincarnation.

47. Reincarnation is an evil concept.

48. I have the will power to accomplish my goals.

49. I am wise enough to make the right choices.

50. I make rational, reasonable choices.

51. I feel love for all other human beings.

52. I bless all other human beings.

53. I bless all who have wronged me.

54. I bless all who have helped me.

55. My life is meaningful.

Copyright C. Norman Shealy, MD, PhD, 2014, Springfield, MO

Reflect on these self-evaluations. There is much to be gained by true introspection!

There is another aspect of personality that must be addressed, and, in my opinion, it is the most critical—Conscientiousness and the NEO (Neuroticism-Extraversion-Openness) Five-Factor Inventory:

Openness to experience—this is the degree of intellectual curiosity, the search for novelty. It generally includes independence, imagination, openness to adventure, art, essentially an eagerness to explore many possibilities.

Conscientiousness includes: organization, responsibility, dependability, industriousness, order, self-control, traditionalism, and virtue. There is considerable evidence that **conscientiousness is the single most critical trait for health, longevity, and even lifetime income.**

Extraversion: outgoing, sociable, prefer stimulation in company of others, more talkative

Agreeableness: More compassionate, trusting, and cooperative

Neuroticism: A tendency to experience unpleasant emotions like anger, anxiety, and depression

Here is a comprehensive way to understand your relation to conscientiousness:

M-CBS Conscientiousness Profile[1]
Circle the number which is most characteristic of YOU!

1. Disagree strongly	5. Agree a little
2. Disagree moderately	6. Agree moderately
3. Disagree a little	7. Agree strongly
4. Neither agree nor disagree	

1---2---3---4---5---6---7	**Prepared**
1---2---3---4---5---6---7	**Neat**
1---2---3---4---5---6---7	**Orderly**
1---2---3---4---5---6---7	**Scheduled**
1---2---3---4---5---6---7	**Focused**
1---2---3---4---5---6---7	**Organized**
1---2---3---4---5---6---7	**Disciplined**
1---2---3---4---5---6---7	**Careful**
1---2---3---4---5---6---7	**Thorough**
1---2---3---4---5---6---7	**Reliable**
1---2---3---4---5---6---7	**Persistent**
1---2---3---4---5---6---7	**Prudent**
1---2---3---4---5---6---7	**Thrifty**
1---2---3---4---5---6---7	**Detailed**
1---2---3---4---5---6---7	**Responsible**
1---2---3---4---5---6---7	**Extrovert**
1---2---3---4---5---6---7	**Prefer Theory**
1---2---3---4---5---6---7	**Logic**
1---2---3---4---5---6---7	**Prefer Facts**

[1]For more information, see http://www.holosenergymedicineeducation.com/M–CB–SCCL.html.

The long eighty-year study on personality and longevity was reported in *The Longevity Project* which was published in 2011. Fifteen hundred 10-year-old children, who were studied and followed for eighty years, proved that conscientiousness was far more important than any other trait for both health and longevity. A network of friends was also tremendously important although not necessarily a distinct part of conscientiousness. Only about 6% of the children were maximally conscientious. It is my impression that over the past sixty years conscientiousness, as measured by Personal Responsibility, has become decreasingly prevalent! When we consider that 40% of Americans are clinically depressed and another 40% are subclinically depressed, at most 20% of Americans appear to have the essential personality for optimal health. As I have emphasized, all emotional problems—from neurotic to psychotic—are the result of low self-esteem and low oxytocin. Therefore, it appears that oxytocin competency is critical for self-esteem, happiness, health, and longevity!

The best way to activate your oxytocin is to use Air Bliss, a blend of essential oils which is applied to thirteen specific acupuncture points. Once you learn the points, it takes only thirty seconds to stimulate the circuit. I have both clinical results of success in 80% of those with depression or anxiety but also laboratory results of the benefits of this approach. You will find more details in my book, *Living Bliss—Major Discoveries along the Holistic Path*. The critical need is to *feel good to yourself!* Once you have optimized your self-nurturing, you are ready to fulfill the only real purpose in life—to help other people!!

First and foremost nurture yourself optimally. You are worth it, and if you take good care of yourself, you will have far more energy to use helping others. So eat, exercise, rest, and exercise optimally. Consider:

Massage
Great music
Tai Chi or Qi Gong
Autogenic Training
Vibratory music
Air Bliss

Join a *Search for God* study group.

Read inspirational books.

Organize your days and weeks. Plan ahead!

Poetry!

Beyond Basics

Here, in alphabetical order, are my recommendations for assisting in many problems:

ADHD

I believe this disorder is grossly overdiagnosed and that Ritalin should be reserved for those who fail to respond to the safe, conservative approach listed below. Furthermore, I think there is *never* an excuse for Prozac® in this situation:

Lithium orotate, 5 to 45 mg daily. 5 mg for 50 pounds, gradually increasing to 45 mg by 150 pounds

Taurine, 1000 to 3000 mg daily

Biogenics® Magnesium Lotion, two teaspoons on skin once or twice daily

Photostimulation with the Shealy RelaxMate II™, an hour daily

Biogenics tapes—start with Basic Schultz daily

Avoid sugar, pop, and aspartame.

If all the above fail, I would use the Shealy PainPro TENS on the Rings of Air and Earth.

EEG biofeedback is also very good but requires one or two sessions a week for six months. I would recommend it only when the above is not effective.

Alcoholism/Addiction

Basics plus:

Ring of Earth stimulation with Air Bliss, plus stimulation of the addiction points, bilaterally.

Lithium orotate, 45 mg daily

Do the *90 Days to Stress-Free Living* program.
If not doing well within one month at the maximum, get past-life
therapy.

Allergies

Most allergies are at least aggravated by food allergies. Start by
avoiding wheat, milk products, eggs, citrus, corn, and peanuts—the most
common food problems.

Add:
- Vitamin D 3, 50,000 units once a week
- K 2, 100 mcg daily.
- Beta-carotene 100,000 to 200,000 units daily
- Astaxanthin, 12 mg daily
- Dr. Shealy's YOUTH Formula, 4 daily—contains 2 grams vitamin C, 1 gram MSM, 6 mg beta 1,3 glucan, and 60 mcg molybdenum
- Vitamin E 400 units daily
- Co-Q 10, 180 mg daily
- Add 2 to 3 tablespoons of chia seeds daily.
- If more is needed, see enhancing Immune Function.

Alzheimer's Disease

Lecithin Granules, two heaping tablespoons twice daily
Stimulation of Ring of Fire daily, **plus** alternate Ring of Air, Earth
and Crystal
Essentials, 2 daily
B 12 at least 1000 mcg, sublingual
Folic acid 100 mg daily
D 3, 50,000 units once a week
Co Q 10, 400 mg daily
Lithium orotate, at least 15 mg daily
Bacopa monnieri, 500 mg, 3 daily
Ashwagandah, 500 mg, 3 daily
Omega-3 fatty acids 3 grams
Cognitol (Om-Chi Herbs) 2 daily
Mem-For (Om-Chi) 3 daily

If not eating ten servings daily, combined, of fruits and veggies:
Tart cherry Juice concentrate, 2 tablespoons daily
A concentrated greens powder, 1 scoop daily
Physical exercise, 1 hour daily

Anxiety/Panic Disorder

Add to basics:
Air Bliss once or twice daily
Double the amount of Biogenics® Magnesium Lotion
Read and practice *90 Days to Stress-Free Living.*
Work Up to Two Hours of Daily Exercise
If not *much* improved in four weeks, add Liss stimulator (Fisher–Wallace) transcranially for one hour each morning and the RelaxMate II an hour at bedtime.
Consider 10 shots of magnesium, IV, if not better in one month.

Arthritis

A majority of arthritis problems are "osteoarthritis." This implies wear and tear and sometimes is the result of trauma. Most of the time it is a metabolic problem, extremely variable, probably to some extent genetically influenced. It may affect just the fingers, or spine, hips, knees, etc. In general, I believe for most people it is the result of inadequate balance between calcium and magnesium, poor Ph balance, excess free radicals, and possibly inadequate water intake over many years.

Try at least two quarts of non–chlorinated, non–fluoridated water daily plus

- Joint Support, one heaping tablespoon and 3 capsules daily
- Boron, 18 mg daily
- Fire Bliss and Earth Bliss daily
- Boswellin, 500 mg three times daily
- Curcumin, same dose. Best to purchase one which also has black pepper or BioPerine
- D 3, 50,000 units once a week. (All these are available at 888–242–6105) *This # has been disconnected*)
- If you must use anti–inflammatory drugs, try aspirin first. Remember, unless you have allergies, L–glutamine may help greatly

with avoiding gastrointestinal complications.

See later for rheumatoid arthritis. There are, of course, many other causes, especially when only one or two joints are affected.

Asthma

Basics plus Anxiety Disorder plus DHEA restoration

Magnesium replacement is essential, especially use of Magnesium Lotion.

Consider food allergy as a contributor—avoid wheat, corn, milk products, eggs, peanuts, and citrus for a month.

Stimulate Ring of Air daily with Shealy Pain Pro TENS.

Autoimmune Diseases:
Lupus, Rheumatoid Arthritis, Scleroderma, Ulcerative colitis, (See Irritable Bowel/Crohn's also), etc.

All the basics plus immune enhancing approaches. The Rings are especially recommended, alternating days with Fire, Earth, and Crystal.

The Seuterman homeopathic approach has also been particularly helpful in scleroderma and rheumatoid arthritis. See below.

Practice the techniques in my book *90 Days to Stress-Free Living*.

Brain Cancer

Certainly I would try 20 IV's of 100 grams of vitamin C in a Myers cocktail, five days a week for four weeks. There are anecdotal reports of cures of six brain tumors. For information contact John Sewell, 706–677–4934. 327 Charity Rd., Homer, Ga. 30547.

Cancer

In general, I do not find most of the somewhat radical "conventional" approaches to help many people. In fact I would **not** use conventional chemotherapy.

I would try:
- My Essentials, 2 per day
- Youth Formula, 4 per day
- Magnesium lotion, 2 teaspoons twice daily

- Vitamin D3, 50,000 units daily. No calcium supplements on this dosage and check serum calcium at three weeks, nine weeks, and then quarterly
- Vitamin K 2, 100 mcg daily
- Co-Q 10, 400 mg daily
- Alfa PXP Royale, build to six scoops daily. Indeed, after six scoops a day for a week or so, I would take fifteen scoops one day.
- Alfa HFI, three daily
- IV vitamin C, 100 grams, in a Myers cocktail, daily, five days a week for at least four weeks
- Castor oil suits nightly for one month
- Saunas five days a week or soak in a bath tub with a cup of magnesium chloride crystals and very warm water for thirty minutes
- Positive mental programming—autogenic training (Basic Schultz CD)
- Rings of Fire and Crystal stimulation (or RejuvaMatrix thirty minutes daily)
- GR 8-Dophilus, 2 twice daily
- Keep your salivary pH at 7.4 to 7.5. Use K–Bicarb if necessary to be alkaline.
- One or two meals of all raw fruits, veggies, nuts, and seeds
- One or two meals of macrobiotic—brown rice, steamed veggies, and broiled, poached or baked fish
- Consult one or two spiritual healers—see list earlier.
- White Bear Double Helix Water
- Consider Protocel.
- Consider heavy enzyme therapy.
- Consider IV or intra-arterial sodium bicarbonate (see *Cancer Is a Fungus* in archived e-newsletters).

One patient cured herself of metastatic cancer to the liver by using abdominal castor oil packs and each night packing the soles of her feet with crushed raw garlic about a cm thick, putting on socks and continuing until the soles of the feet blistered after about five days! I followed her "cure" after that for at least five years, and I then lost track of her.

Actually, personally I would use the RejuvaMatrix ™ one hour daily.

Candidiasis/Yeast Infections Vaginally

All basics plus Enhancing Immune Function

There have been several published reports showing that a 600 mg vaginal suppository of boric acid provides symptomatic relief in just twenty-four hours. It usually takes about ten days of treatment (one 600 mg suppository capsule inserted in the morning and another in the evening) to wipe out the infection. If the problem returns, a repeated course of treatment of two to three days might be needed.

One study compared boric acid suppositories to the common drug nystatin. Boric acid was far superior, with a 92% cure rate compared to a 64% cure rate with nystatin. (Journal of Acquired Immune Deficiency Syndrome and Human Retrovirology 97; 16(3): 219-220.) Both the capsules and the boric acid are available at pharmacies.

Also see in my newsletter archives *Cancer Is a Fungus*.

Carpal Tunnel Syndrome

At least half the patients who have been told they have this do not. An accurate diagnosis is possible only with a sensory nerve conduction study. Smokers have CTS at least twice as often as non-smokers. At least 80% of the time, in non-smokers, the following is curative:

Massage the wrist twice daily with a mixture of equal parts of emu and castor oil. Do passive extension of the hand for five minutes.

Take 1000 mg B6 for one month, 500 mg for one month, and 100 mg thereafter. **Do not** continue the larger dosages beyond that second month!

Use magnesium lotion on the skin, anywhere, two teaspoons twice daily.

Extension stretches of the hand twice daily
Earth Bliss twice daily

Cholesterol/Coronary Artery Disease

There is no circumstance under which I would take any of the cholesterol lowering drugs (statins). They are dangerous, and it is another experiment like PremPro® that may not be revealed until thousands have suffered complications and/or death.

What to do?

Avoid like the plague all margarines and artificially hardened fats.

So, my latest recommendations for optimal cholesterol (160 to 180; *not below* 150 HDL *at least* 40 TO 60):

- Do not take statins.

- Keep your weight between 19 and 24 body mass index.

- Eat wisely, avoiding junk and junk fast food, hydrogenated fats, excess carbs.

- Exercise wisely, at least an hour a day.

- Relax and practice stress reduction.

- D 3, 50,000 units once a week

- Use only butter, olive oil, and flax seed oils as added fats.

- If you are a man by age 50 take at least 1200 mg of beta sitosterol complex—up to 4200 mg to keep the prostate healthy or saw palmetto double strength extract, 160 mg, 8 to 12 daily.

- In women, add at least 1200 mg of beta sitosterol complex and up to 4200 mg.

- If that does not work, add lecithin granules, two heaping tablespoons twice daily.

- If that does not work, add Kyani NitroXtreme, 15 to 30 drops twice daily.

Avoid homogenized milk. That makes the fat much more dangerous.

Drink plenty of real water—not chlorinated/fluoridated.

Eat lots of fruits and veggies.

Have your homocysteine level checked; it is ten times as important and easily controlled with extra B 12 and folic acid.

Chronic fatigue/fibromyalgia
(See also Electromagnetic Dysthymia)

Use the complete Anxiety and Depression Regimens, plus DHEA Restoration and Adrenal Fatigue.

Comprehensive management for chronic pain and difficult diseases—including failed back surgery, thalamic pain syndrome, post–herpetic neuralgia, etc. Always the Shealy PainPro TENS first, including the Ring of Earth. If that is inadequate, then:

A competent, charismatic, compassionate, holistic physician, who selects the team and uses:

No use of mood or pain drugs

Cranial Electrical Stimulation

SheLi TENS™

Biofeedback, autogenic training, and related self–regulation techniques

Massage

Heat and cold

Hot tubs

Vibratory music beds

Acupuncture

Humanistic psychological approaches

Good nutrition, including supplements

Physical exercise, including yoga and free form tai chi

IV magnesium chloride in a Myers cocktail, at least 10 doses

Depression (including bipolar)

Add to basics plus Anxiety suggestions:

1. Meat broth: 8 oz. of stew–sized meat, cooked overnight in slow-cooker, low heat, with 1 quart water, 2 tablespoons vinegar and seasonings to taste. Drink at least 2 cups daily.
2. Photostimulation: Use the Shealy RelaxMate II at least 40 to 60 minutes daily.
3. Use the LISS TENS transcranially for 40 to 60 minutes daily or use Fire .
4. Listen to great classical music at least one hour daily.
5. If not doing well after a month, add Lithium Orotate, 45 mg daily (Bipolars should start with this).
6. Tryptophan, 1000 mg and up to at least 5000 mg per day is actually wonderful for most depressed people.

DHEA Restoration

There are four excellent techniques for restoration of DHEA, highly recommended. Unless you have a serious disease such as lupus, I do not recommend taking DHEA supplements. And do not ever take DHEA supplements if you have cancer of prostate, breast, uterus, or ovaries.

The four techniques, all safe, and work independently of each other, each adding to the other:

1. Ring of Fire Stimulation with the Shealy PainPro TENS™. Obviously you could use acupuncture, but it is much less expensive in the long run to buy the stimulator and use it.

2. Natural Progesterone (Eugesterone) cream, ¼ tsp twice daily on the skin. For men, use Adam's Prostate Care.

3. Dr. Shealy's Youth Formula, 4 daily

4. Biogenics® Magnesium Lotion, 4 to 6 tsp on skin daily

Diabetes

Add to basics:

Weight must be within 18 to 24 Body Mass Index!!!!

Tri-Chromium, 1000 micrograms

Gugulipid, 250 mg, 3 daily

Gymnema, 250 mg, 3 daily

Zinc picolinate, 50 mg

Alpha Lipoic Acid, 500 mg twice daily

Exercise and follow the advice in *90 Days to Stress-Free Living!*

Those on insulin or antidiabetic meds must exercise caution in using Gugulipid and Gymnema, as these can lower blood sugar. I would recommend these only with careful monitoring of blood sugars, preferably under the direction of a holistically oriented physician or nurse practitioner.

Eczema

This condition is almost always associated with allergies to some food. Avoid coffee, wheat, milk products, eggs, citrus, corn products, peanuts, and chocolate for a month. If it improves markedly, add one food at a time, each week to determine which must be eliminated long-term.

Add evening primrose oil and fish oil capsules—total of 6 to 12 grams.

Try lecithin granules, two tablespoons twice daily.

Vitamin E 400 units

Daily saunas may help but need several months to be sure of results.

Electromagnetic Dysthymia (Chronic Fatigue; Fibromyalgia)

EMD is a generalized disorder of chronic fatigue, anxiety, depression, and a significantly weakened immune system. It is rarely diagnosed and goes under the rubric of environmental allergies, candidiasis, chronic fatigue, M–E (in England), REDD syndrome, etc. All these problems are associated with deficiency in DHEA, magnesium, and essential amino acids, especially Tryptophan and Taurine.

This problem is the most difficult one I know other than cancer! It takes three months of intense therapy.

- Daily use of the Liss Cranial Electrical Stimulator (now sold as Fisher–Wallace) one hour between 9 AM and noon
- Twice daily use of Air Bliss on the Ring of Air
- Daily use of the Shealy PainPro on the Ring of Fire
- 10 to 15 IVs of 2 grams magnesium chloride in Myers cocktail
- Daily use of magnesium lotion
- Daily use of the Shealy RelaxMate for one hour at bedtime
- My Youth Formula 4 daily
- For most people Eugesterone twice daily. Men use Adam's prostate care.
- Beef broth daily or add tryptophan 2000 mg and taurine 2000 mg daily

Endometriosis

Keep your body mass index below 25!

Use Eugesterone cream from day 10 to day 28 of cycle, or start of next cycle.

Stress reduction

Enhancing Immune Function

All basics plus
All DHEA Restoration as above, plus daily:
Vitamin D 3, 50,000 units once a week
Double Helix Water added to non–chlorinated water
Vitamin K 2 100 mcg daily

Glutamine powder, 2 tablespoons daily
Alfa PXP Royale, 1 to 3 scoops daily
Co Q10 400 mg daily
Maxogenol, 4 daily
Coconut oil, 3 tablespoons daily
Castor Oil packs to the abdomen or baths
Autogenic training (Basic Schultz CD)
In severe problems, IVs daily for 10 to 20 days of 100 grams of vitamin C in a Myers cocktail
90 Days to Stress-Free Living, the book/program by me

Five Sacred Rings

Over the past ten years I have discovered in the human body five circuits, which activate specific chemical pathways. The stimulation required appears to be that of either the LISS TENS® or the Shealy PainPro TENS™. In general the PainPro is more effective. For those individuals who are very sensitive to electrical current, the Liss may be more easily accepted. The Liss puts out 15,000 pulses per second, modulated 15 and 500 times per second. The Shealy puts out all frequencies, including 54 to 78 billion pulses per second. This latter frequency is that which has been proven by Ukrainian physicists to equal the frequency of human DNA. Regular TENS and the AlphaStim® did not raise DHEA.

The circuits are:

Fire: which increases DHEA, the adrenal hormone that is low or deficient in most individuals because of excess stress. In addition to raising DHEA, stimulation of **Fire** has been clinically successful in 70 to 80% of patients who have rheumatoid arthritis, migraine, depression or diabetic neuropathy. Stimulation must be done daily for three months and then at least twice a week to maintain the improvement. Points: K 3; CV 2, 6 and 18; B 22; MH6; LI 18; GV 20. The Shealy PainPro TENS is the only one that works in diabetic neuropathy.

Water: which optimizes aldosterone, the hormone responsible for regulation of water and potassium. Theoretically it may help balance emotions. Combined with **Fire**, stimulation of **Water** and **Fire** has been found to help significantly in weight loss. The points are: Sp 4; GV 8, 20; CV 14; B 10, 13; H 7; TH 16.

Air: which raises neurotensin, a neurochemical which helps fat metabolism but is also a neuroleptic. This effect appears to assist in establishing a meditative state or "simultaneity of thought." Points are Sp 1a; LIV 3; S 36, 9; B 60; LI 16; GV 20.

Earth: which raises calcitonin significantly. Calcitonin is a hormone produced in the thyroid and is the key regulator of calcium metabolism in bone. Calcitonin is a powerful tool for maintaining strong bones. Calcitonin is also forty to sixty times as strong as morphine in reducing pain. Stimulation of this ring may help addiction, ground the personality, and be an adjunct in rebuilding the body. Points: K 1; B 60, 54; LI 16; S 9; SI 17; GV 20.

Crystal: which reduces free radicals significantly, within three days of starting daily stimulation, especially with the SheLi TENS. Free radicals are the destructive chemicals that cause aging and degeneration. Theoretically, reducing free radicals could be the single most important adjunct for enhancing health and longevity. The Shealy PainPro TENS is best. Points are: SP 4; G 11, 30.5; CV 8.5, 14.5, 23; GV 4.5, 7.5, 14.5, 20.

Fibromyalgia—See Electromagnetic Dysthymia.

Growth Hormone Activation/Anti-Aging

1. *I do not recommend* growth hormone itself.
2. Peak exercise—build to 30 seconds of the fastest you can do of any exercise to breathing exhaustion, 8 times with 90 seconds of rest after each 30 second set. Do this at least 3 and not more than 4 times a week!
3. Royal maca up to one tablespoon daily has some excellent evidence for overall rejuvenation, including sometimes controlling all menopausal symptoms. A small number of people develop hypertension on maca.
4. Regular use of Biogenics® Magnesium Lotion
5. For men, Tribulus, 500 mg, 4 to 8 daily to help restore testosterone production
6. Wear a Clarus Q-Pendant. It protects you from 50 milligaus of EMF (888-242-6105).

Hepatitis C

Actually there are basics for all hepatitis, especially the acute phase. Ideally IVs of 50 to 100 grams of vitamin C, with calcium, magnesium, B 6, etc. Actually Myers cocktail with boosted C.
All the immune enhancing approaches.
Add milk thistle, 500 mg 3 or 4 daily.
RejuvaMatrix™ one hour daily

Hypertension

Add to basics:
Double the amount of Biogenics® Magnesium Lotion.
Kyani NitroXtreme, 15 to 30 drops twice daily
Body mass Index **must** be 18 to 24.
Calcium citrate or coral calcium 1000 mg daily
D 3, 50,000 units once a week
Learn to warm feet to 96 degrees mentally!
Read and practice *90 Days to Stress-Free Living.*
Co-Q 10, 200 to 300 mg daily
Omega 3 Fatty acids, 4000 to 6000 mg daily
Taurine, 6000 mg daily

Headache

See Migraine. In general, once competent medical evaluation has ruled out any other problem, most headaches will respond to the approaches for migraine.

Hyperthyroidism

Eat broccoli, kale, cauliflower, cabbage, etc. daily.
Lithium Orotate, 45 mg daily
Lemon Balm as tea or tincture, 4 times daily
Bugleweed, as tea or tincture , 4 times daily
Shealy RelaxMate—use at least 20 minutes three times a day.
Autogenic training—Basic Schultz CD twice daily
Castor oil packs to thyroid
Double the basic dose of Biogenics® Magnesium Lotion.

Avoid caffeine, aspartame, etc.

Hypothyroidism

Iodoral one daily for 4 to 6 weeks. Fire Bliss daily

Impotentia

Always start with saw palmetto extract, 160 mg, double strength extract, 4 to 8 daily and pygeum, 50 mg, 4 daily.

If there is no severe vascular disease or neuropathy, then the following may be useful:

Tribulus, 500 mg, up to 8 daily

DHEA restoration as above

Epimedium sagittatum, 100 mg, up to 6 daily

TestoJack 200, 2 daily which adds:

Xanthoparmelia scabrosa, Cnidium monnier

If all else fails, and you are not on antihypertensive medication, consider Tadalafil.

Insomnia

All basics plus:

LISS TENS transcranially one hour daily

Shealy RelaxMate II, one hour as you fall asleep

Taurine 3000 mg at bedtime

Melatonin timed release, 1 mg up to 10 mg at bedtime

Lithium orotate, 45 mg at bedtime

If not effective, switch to:

Tryptophan, build up to 10 grams, but continue lithium orotate and 2 Dr. Shealy's Essentials

All of these are available at 888-242-6105.

If these fail, consider LifeWave Silent Nights.

Irritable Bowel/Leaky Gut/Crohn's Disease

Avoid wheat, corn, citrus, eggs, dairy, peanuts, chocolate, aspartame, junk food, and pop.

Start with glutamine powder, one teaspoon with each meal.

Glucan, one teaspoon with each meal
Vitamin D 3, 50,000 units once a week
K 2, 100 micrograms daily
DS–8 Dophilus, 5 caps daily
Formula 29, one tablespoon daily
If not better in a week, try folic acid 100 mg daily.
Intestinalis, 4 daily
Boswellin, 250 mg, 4 daily, available at 888–242–6105.

If not much better in a another week, stop Boswellin and add Hanna Kroger's Wormwood Combination, 4 daily and add 2 daily building to 12 daily for one month.

Avoid all *gluten* products.

Deal with your unfinished emotional hang–ups!!!

Macular Degeneration

All the usual, plus immune enhancing approaches, as this is clearly a disease of excess free radicals and inadequate antioxidants.

Most important, daily:
Chelated Zinc, 30 mg
Taurine, 3000 mg
 Co Q 10, 300 mg
Beta carotene, 25,000 units
Astaxanthin, 30 mg
Vitamin E, 400 units
Youth Formula, 4

In addition, there is good evidence that electrical stimulation, with the Liss TENS, of the closed eyes, 10 minutes daily is of benefit if started early.

I'd also recommend stimulation at least of the Ring of Fire and Ring of Crystal *with* Shealy PainPro.

Meniere's Syndrome

Always basics with plenty of magnesium. Try avoiding wheat, milk products, citrus, egg, corn, chocolate, peanuts.

Food allergies may be a major contributor.

Cocculus, a homeopathic remedy may help

Acupuncture is one option.

Finally stimulation of the Ring of Air with Air Bliss

Menopausal Symptoms

Add to basics:

Start with natural progesterone cream, EUGESTERONE, ¼ tsp twice daily on the skin.

If ovaries have been removed or symptoms not controlled, *try* vaginal Estriol cream.

If you are on PremPro® and want to come off:

Start with the Eugesterone cream and after 3 weeks cut your PremPro dose in half. In another 3 weeks go to every other day. After another 3 weeks go to every third day. In another three weeks, stop PremPro. If you have hot flashes, add Herbal-F, three daily. This product contains the effective herbal pro-estrogens.

If the herbal preparation does not work, then you need a prescription, to be filled at a compounding pharmacy, containing in a daily total dose of two ¼ tsp 60 mg of natural progesterone and 2.5 mg of biest (estriol and estradiol). I do not recommend estrone. Rarely testosterone may be needed also and may be added to the cream.

Do autogenic training—Basic Schultz CD.

The Methuselah Promise—Healthy Youthing

In addition to the Ring of Fire, stimulation of the Rings of Crystal and Earth should optimize overall health and longevity. When you add all five Rings, there is significant evidence of telomere regeneration—the single best indication of improved longevity and health!

Migraine

Add to basics:

1. Temperature biofeedback. Those who *learn* to raise temperature of the index finger to 96 degrees mentally within 5 minutes reduce severity and frequency by 84%.

2. Ring of Fire: Stimulation daily with the Shealy PainPro TENS reduces frequency by 75%—almost twice as good as the "best"

drug for prophylaxis, Depakote, which has **many** complications. Indeed, I will not recommend that drug.

3. Posture Pump is superb. See my newsletter archives.
4. Computerized cervical traction: Daily for two weeks. Excellent adjunct and reduces or eliminates many types of headache.
5. The Shealy RelaxMate II used 20 minutes three times a day is helpful to many patients. There is no better relaxation device for relaxation!
6. Autogenic training, even without biofeedback is tremendously useful.
7. Food sensitivities: Two-thirds of migraineurs reduce frequency markedly by avoiding wheat, corn, eggs, citrus, milk products, peanuts, chocolate, red wine, cheese, pickled herring. After 6 weeks or so, if headaches are markedly improved, add back one of these food groups each week to see which must be permanently avoided
8. **No** aspartame; no smoking; no pop.
9. Biogenics® Magnesium Lotion, 2 teaspoons twice daily. All migraineurs are deficient in magnesium.
10. Riboflavin, vitamin B2, 400 mg daily is helpful in some patients.
11. Natural progesterone cream, ¼ tsp on skin twice daily from 10 to 28th day of cycle or until next cycle begins, whichever is earliest.
12. Get and do my book *90 Days to Stress-Free Living.*
13. Tryptophan 1000 mg 3 or 4 times daily plus 45 mg of lithium orotate is often helpful.
14. Taurine 1000 mg, three times daily may be helpful.
15. Avoid MSG—fast foods and Asian restaurants load this toxin in their foods.

Multiple Sclerosis, ALS, etc.

Multiple Sclerosis Diet
Avoid wheat and gluten!!
Vitamin D 3, 50,000 units once a week
Use all the immune enhancing tools plus Fire, Earth, and Crystal Bliss.

Obesity

Always check your temperature before getting out of bed. If it is consistently below 97.6, you have relative hypothyroidism. Iodoral one daily for a month may help. If not, add the Ring of Fire and the Ring of Water, stimulated with Shealy PainPro TENS.

In general, the Barnes diet works best for most people. It consists of maximum of two servings of bread and one small serving of fruit total per day plus unlimited eggs, meat of all kinds and non-starchy veggies.

For those recalcitrant to Barnes, the rice diet is recommended—unlimited rice and canned fruits! Repulsive after a while but it works!

Or two meals daily of raw fruits, veggies, nuts and seeds and one of brown rice, broiled or baked fish and steamed veggies.

Increase your exercise slowly over several months to at least one hour daily.

Finally the Rings of Fire and Water with Bliss oils each day may help.

Attitude and activity are essential! And *no* aspartame.

Obsessive Compulsive Disorder

Before going on drugs, do the basics, plus anxiety, plus depression regimen and add Lithium Orotate, 45 mg daily.

Tryptophan, 1000 mg three to four times daily

Osteoporosis

Earth Bliss daily

Eugesterone, ¼ tsp on skin twice a day or Adam's Prostate care for men

Biogenics® Magnesium Lotion, two teaspoons twice a day on skin

Boron, 12 mg daily

Vitamin D 3, 50,000 units once a week

Exercise—a minimum of 30 minutes daily!

PMS

Eugesterone cream, ¼ tsp twice daily from day 10 until day 28 or start of next period

Zinc 30 mg daily
B 6 100 mg daily
Lots of physical exercise
Basic Schultz CD daily

Prostate Problems (BPH or Cancer)

Always Basics plus:
Drink at least 2 quarts of good water daily
Vitamin D 3 , 50,000 units once a week
Vitamin K 2, 100 mcg daily
C0-Q 10–at least 300 mg daily. 600 mg if you have cancer.
Quercetin, 250 mg, 4 daily
Take small flower willow tea, 3 cups daily, for at least two weeks yearly and up to 6 weeks if you have symptoms.
Saw palmetto, double strength extract, 160 mg, 6 to 12 daily, depending on intensity of symptoms
Start with these above. If symptoms are not markedly improved within 4 to 6 weeks, add:
 Pygeum, 50 mg. Two to 10 daily
Nettles capsules, 2 twice daily
Cernilton, 4 to 6 daily
With cancer, use Immune Enhancement.
Stay sexually active! Use it at least 2 or 3 times a week or lose it! If you do not have a partner, masturbate and enjoy it.
In chronic prostatitis, but not cancer, prostate massage at least 3 times weekly.

Rosacea

Basics plus:
Enhancing Immune Function plus
Try eliminating wheat, corn, eggs, dairy citrus, chocolate, and peanuts for one month. If you improve add one food at a time, one a week, to see if there is a specific.
Apply emu oil to skin twice daily. If that does not work, try jojoba oil.

Psoriasis

All the usual health enhancing approaches.

This autoimmune disease of the skin often responds very well to a diet of two meals daily of raw vegetables, fruits, seeds, and nuts. The third meal should be broiled or baked fish with steamed vegetables and brown rice. Use a tablespoon or two of raw flax seed oil over the veggies and /or rice.

D 3, 50,000 units once a week

K 2 15 mg daily

Biogenics® Magnesium Lotion—apply on **normal** skin only.

Take Essentials, Co-Q 10 at least 120 mg daily and 6 grams Omega 3 Fatty Acids.

Avoid wheat and gluten like the plague!!

Seuterman homeopathy may be helpful.

Seuterman Homeopathy

This approach uses 6 homeopathic agents each treatment:

Traditional homeopathic

Nosode

Krebs cycle

Quinone

Detox

Organ tissue

If you are interested in my protocol for rheumatoid and autoimmune diseases, email me with a request at norm@normshealy.com.

Shingles

If started early, either amantadine or ramantadine is worth trying, with daily, at least 6 grams of vitamin C, 100 mg of B Complex, lysine 3000 mg and zinc 100 mg, and vitamin D 3, 3000 units.

Once postherpetic shingles pain starts, the treatment of choice is the Shealy PainPro TENS with electrodes above and below the scar. If that does not work, try the Ring of Earth.

Uterine Fibroids

In general this problem is the result of long years of estrogen dominance. It is best treated with natural progesterone cream, Eugesterone, ¼ tsp twice daily on the skin from the 10th to the 28th day of cycle or start of next cycle.

Secondly, keep your weight at 18 to 24 BMI. Fatty tissue contributes estrogen!

Exercise vigorously, building up to equivalent of 4 miles of brisk walking in 1 hour at least 5 days a week.

Castor oil packs on the abdomen daily for at least a month

Stimulation of the Ring of Fire with Fire Bliss

You might consult a healer. This is the type of problem that may respond to spiritual healing.

8

Soul, Spirit, Religion, and Meditation

I have never had difficulty understanding soul—to me it is the essence of each individual on its unique journey to adequate perfection in some life so that it can "return" to God. I cannot even begin to understand what that ultimate return really is or even what God is. I have unequivocal faith that there is a benevolent Supreme Power that somehow created all that is. To me religion, virtually always, is a fight for God—each religion somehow strives to prove that it is the only truth, and in that fight they all miss the mark! Ultimately, the search for God is the role of true meditation—attunement with soul, spirit, and God or the Divine. Allegorically I see the soul as the puppeteer, the entity that chooses each life, with the intent of correcting a life experience. The soul is the "developing" part of the individual. Once the soul has selected two parents, the experience is almost like a slot machine—not that I even vaguely understand slot machines! But, the choice of parents, who have two remarkably variable sets of genes, can theoretically lead to a combination of about a trillion different mixes. With that push of

199

the button on the slot machine, the genes contain the memories of all the ancestors of both parents, and I believe, somewhere in that matrix, the Akashic records of the individual soul incarnating. I believe that almost invariably the incarnating soul has some previous lifetime of connection with both parents. Nevertheless, the new parents may or may not be optimally nurturing, kind, supportive, etc. Even before the conception, the health of either parent may not be optimal and may be potentially harmful to the new fetus, because of the unique habits of each parent. The thoughts, actions, and behaviors, especially of the mother during fetal life profoundly affect the future child, as does the entire circumstance around birth. Then there are the critical first seven years of life which appear to affect self-esteem, beliefs, and values more than anything else measurable.

Some souls carry greater wisdom and resiliency or stamina, and the parental environment can help or hinder the new life. Thousands of events in the maturing life set the stage for the further challenges and success of the individual. Cayce referred frequently to astrological influences, and I have been intrigued by astrology since at least age 16. To me the most influential aspects are the Sun, Moon, Ascendant or Rising, and the North Node.

Sun:
- Aries—Fearlessly naïve and forcefully direct, audacious, and of course fiery
- Taurus—Ferdinand the bull is a perfect allegory—strong, peaceful, artistic but don't sting him on the buttocks!
- Gemini—Versatile and rapidly changeable, mercurial indeed.
- Cancer—I prefer Moon Child—More than any other sign, Cancer personality mood is highly tied to phases of the moon. Imaginative and strongly emotional.
- Leo—Rulers of the world. There are more Leo's in positions of authority than all other signs combined! Commanding and regal
- Virgo—Perfectionists, organizers, dependable, and sincere. The ultimate conscientious person
- Libra—Intelligent, doves of peace who like justice and fairness above all, but often have trouble making a decision because of the need to be fair.

- Scorpio—Intelligent, authoritarian, controlling, highly sexed
- Sagittarius—Blunt—foot in mouth, honest, idealist, idiosyncratic
- Capricorn—ambitious, serious, persistent
- Aquarius—a butterfly chasing a rainbow, wide interests, team player
- Pisces—Masters of satire, highly intuitive, sensitive

These few attributes for each sun sign are tremendously modified by some of **the same 12 signs** being placed dominantly in **Rising Sign/ Ascendant** which is the influence the individual wants the world to see, and by the **Moon** which significantly influences the emotions of the individual, and by the **North Node** which represents the major challenges of this life.

And of course there are other significant influences in relation to the placement of Jupiter, Uranus, Saturn, Mars, etc.! The dominant influences of these planets at birth are further modified by the movement of these planets at varying speeds throughout life. The astrological influences can be as strong as the many genetic and karmic ones!

In a given life, the individual—entity—gains or loses the higher human potentials, and each overall human lifetime is a remarkable part of the soul's experience.

Cayce saw the life force itself as the spirit, which is always perfect, made in the image of God. All spirits are the universal collective mind of God and part of the "oneness of God." At a soul level, once the individual is incarnated, the mind of the individual is the builder! It has free will, and the body is the result of the overall mind of the individual. The spirit is always aware of its identity with God, while the soul knows only what it has experienced. When the will of the soul becomes no different from the essence of God, the soul returns to spirit—at one with God.

According to Cayce,

G.34   4/27/38   [Emphasis is the author's.]

While each soul, each associate, each acquaintance *is* an obligation, a duty — all of these must cooperate, coordinate. As the

body itself in its welfare, mentally or physically, unless it cooperates, coordinates each portion with the other, there is not the
well-rounded, the well-balanced individual nor the better and
best reactions from same.

There is the physical body, there is the mental body, there
is the spiritual body. They are one. They each have their attributes. They each have their weaknesses. They each have their
associations. Yet they must be all coordinated

Meditation

In general, meditation is the most powerful tool for moving the
individual towards the true divine spirit and union with God. And
there are many roads to Rome and God. Quieting the idle chatter of the
mind—mindfulness—is essential. This can involve music, singing, chant-
ing, dancing, walking, breathing, and focused affirmations. No one can
take you into meditation. You can take yourself there or be guided to
the foothills of meditation, but true meditation is the attunement with
God/Divine. As indicated earlier, autogenic training(AT) can condition
the mind and body to be at peace, balanced and those who do AT regularly will after six months often begin to have spontaneous spiritual
images. And significant self-regulation technique assists in helping one
achieve the meditative state. And as emphasized earlier, balancing body
sensations and emotions is a major prerequisite. Then spiritual uplifting
music and images may help you across the threshold and beyond the
foothills. One of my favorite images of the soul came from Dr. Robert
Leichtman over thirty years ago—a five-pointed sky-blue star. He then
gave a favorite image for God—a giant white six-pointed star, beaming down on the Universe a magnificent golden-orange light. Golden
globes, golden pyramids, angels, etc. may be part of the imagery.

In his *Allegory of the Cave* Plato likened the senses of the body to
entering the cave. The senses are the chains that make us prisoners to
the multidimensional higher spiritual world. The prisoner's journey to
enlightenment is the way out of the cave. In the *Allegory of the Chariot*,
the reason and intellect of the personality/soul are the charioteer, as
the chariot is driven by a winged mortal horse and a winged immortal
horse. Essentially there is a battle between the two winged horses, so

that when they approach the threshold of heaven, they clash and fall back to earth to recuperate and start the race over. The road to enlightenment/truth may go from the lowest to the highest representation of the charioteer—tyrant, demagogue, craftsman/farmer, poet, prophet, health practitioner, politician/manager/business person, honest law-abiding King or Ruler, to the ultimate philosopher—one who is dedicated to beauty and love.

Once again, I am taken back to Assagioli's concept:

> I have a mind and I am much more than mind.
> I have a body and I am much more than body.
> I have sensations and I am much more than sensations.
> I have emotions and I am much more than emotions.
> At my innermost level I am **magnificent, wise and loving!!**
> This is the journey to enlightenment!! And meditation is a major part of the journey.

Incidentally, this is a key exercise to do as a regular reminder to detach from the stress and strain of the outer world! With all exercises, begin by assuming a comfortable position—sitting with legs crossed is excellent. If that is not comfortable, recline with a bolster under your knees. Close your eyes and begin by taking a few slow deep breaths. Preparation for meditation requires that you release from your focus of attention **all** negative distractions. Thus, it is important to practice, practice, practice examining your body, mind, emotions and attitudes and releasing **all** anger, fear, anxiety, guilt, and sadness over anything. Gradually your entire being is trained to be at peace and ready for attunement with your soul and with God.

Releasing Tension

Assume a comfortable position and begin by taking a few slow deep breaths. Then as you breathe in, scan your feet and legs and collect any tension with your breath. Then exhale, releasing the tension.

Repeat.

Next breath, scan your pelvis, collect the tension—exhale, releasing the tension.

Repeat

Next breath, scan your abdomen, collect the tension—exhale, releasing the tension.

Repeat

Next breath, scan your chest, collect the tension—exhale, releasing the tension.

Repeat

Next breath, scan your neck, shoulders, arms, and hands, collect the tension—exhale, releasing the tension.

Repeat

Next breath, scan you entire head and mind, collect the tension—exhale, releasing the tension.

Repeat

Next breath, scan you entire body, toes to head, collect any residual tension—exhale, releasing the tension.

Repeat

Now you are **ready** for meditation! Allow your mind to focus on your soul. Create a magnificent sky-blue five-pointed star, a metaphor for your soul. Merge with the star. Stay as long as you like and return to your regular life by taking a deep closing breath, releasing it, and opening your eyes.

Focusing Your Heartbeat

Every cell in your body pulsates with every heartbeat. After beginning with a few initial relaxing breaths, allow yourself to feel the pulsations of your heartbeat in your lips. Spend whatever time you like enjoying this sensation but **never** allow yourself to feel the pulsations inside your head. If you suddenly find yourself there, quickly switch and feel the pulsations **only** in your hands! Then explore your ability to *feel* the pulsations in your neck, pausing a few moments in each area. Then your chest—abdomen—pelvis—feet, etc. Finish the exercise by focusing love and appreciation on your heart.

Joy

Start by recalling the happiest, most loving event of your entire life. Relive the experience. Then as you continue to re-experience joy, just say quietly to yourself *joy* as you breathe in and *joy* as you breathe out. Continue as long as you like and allow yourself to feel and experience true *joy*.

Life Lessons

What are your life lessons? Might they be patience, detachment, forgiveness, tolerance, serenity? After entering your deepest possible state of relaxation, focus on just one word—repeating it as you breathe in and breathe out. If your mind wanders, just return to the word and **see** the experience. This one is worth many sessions!

Solutions

Before you begin, recognize a problem. Then relax and ask yourself:
Is this a problem I can solve with actions, by words, or physically?
If not, then ask: Can I divorce this problem? Just move away from it and release it.
If not, am I ready to forgive it? Release it into the hands of God.

Blessings

After relaxing well, begin to think of all those who have helped you in some way. Start with your parents! No matter what your over-all relationship with them is/was, they gave you life. Bless them with images and words—and especially with **meaning**! Then consider other family members, teachers, friends, spouse, children, etc. This could be **many** sessions!

Thoughts

After relaxing, focus on feeling the meaning of these words:
Every thought is a prayer. Thinking sets in motion spiritual forces to

bring about change in body, mind, attitudes, hopes, and despairs. Be aware throughout each day: Are my thought creating **joy**?

Love

After relaxing focus on this phrase:
Love is the *desire to do good to—to help—others!*

Faith

No matter what happens, **faith** means that you believe the purpose in life is **good** and that ultimately **good** will come out of every challenge. After relaxing, just focus on **faith** with every breath in and every breath out. Sense, see, feel **faith**!

Hope

No matter the situation, there is always **hope** that the future will be better. After relaxing, focus on every breath in and every breath out on the word **hope**. Sense, see, feel **hope**!

What else is needed?

What else is needed—patience, virtue, tranquility, peace, responsibility, power, wealth, meaning? Each of these and many other such words are worth many sessions similar to those above! Spend whatever time is needed to bring yourself into harmony with every word and thought!!!!

More Introspections:

Emotions
What do emotions mean to you? On a scale of zero to ten, how much do you feel:
- Anger
- Anxiety
- Fear

- Guilt
- Depression

What physical feelings/symptoms do these memories create? What unfinished business do you have with each of these? Are you ready to deal with all of it? Do you need to speak with anyone about any of these? Are you ready to release all of them and move on?

Love Your Body

After five minutes of slow, relaxing breathing, tune into your body, feel your

Face/Jaws

Neck and throat

Shoulders, arms, and hands

Chest and breasts

Heart

Lungs

Abdomen, and each organ—stomach, intestines, liver, spleen, kidneys, bladder

Pelvis—sexual organs

Back, spine

Buttocks

Thighs, calves, and feet

If there is any tightness, discomfort, pain, or **no feeling**, be aware that something is out of balance! Talk to the part, love it, thank it!

Attitude

Evelyn Underhill, a great mystic, said "Living the spiritual life is the attitude you hold in your mind when you are down on your knees scrubbing the steps."

What is your attitude?

- On awakening
- When you greet the first person you see, including seeing yourself in the mirror
- As you dress, use the bathroom, prepare for the day
- As you eat each meal
- Throughout all your work or activities of the day

- As you reflect back on the day
- As you bathe
- As you prepare for sleep
- What is the **meaning** of your life??

Power

Caroline Myss has said that the purpose in life is to learn to use power wisely, responsibility, and lovingly. Power is your inner reserve, your feeling of personal control, your thinking, your actions, and your feelings. It is freedom from anger, anxiety, guilt, and depression. Power is having confidence, the willingness to make choices, to choose healthy habits, to set and to achieve goals, to feel yourself in harmony with your Higher Self—your soul!

Archetypes

My archetypes are Child, Victim, Saboteur, Prostitute (we all share these four), Healer, Hero, Warrior, Judge, Visionary, Mystic, Puck, Sage.

Casting my earliest charts, these archetypes fit in the houses in my charts in these very different ways:

One of the keys to understanding yourself and life in general is archetypes. These then interact with twelve different aspect of life.

My Archetypes

Each archetype manifests itself physically (Tribal), emotionally (Individual), or symbolically (as a metaphor)

Career
1. Visionary—Symbolic
2. Healer—Tribal
3. Puck—S
4. Prostitute—T
5. Saboteur—S
6. Hero—Individual
7. Sage—I

8. Victim—I
9. Mystic—I
10. Judge—I
11. Child—I
12. Warrior—S

Family

1. Child—I
2. Mystic—T
3. Puck—S
4. Hero—I
5. Prostitute—T
6. Visionary—S
7. Saboteur—I
8. Judge—S
9. Victim—S
10. Warrior—S
11. Healer—T
12. Sage—T

Finances

1. Hero—S
2. Victim—I
3. Healer—I
4. Mystic—I
5. Prostitute—T
6. Visionary—I
7. Sage—I
8. Puck—I
9. Judge—T
10. Warrior—I
11. Saboteur—S
12. Child—S

Sexuality

1. Puck—T
2. Hero—I

3. Victim—I
4. Sage—S
5. Judge—I
6. Saboteur—I
7. Warrior—T
8. Healer—T
9. Prostitute—I
10. Mystic—S
11. Child—I
12. Visionary—S

Personal Power
1. Victim—S
2. Hero—S
3. Healer—T
4. Sage—T
5. Saboteur—S
6. Puck—S
7. Child—T
8. Judge—I
9. Prostitute—T
10. Warrior—I
11. Mystic—T
12. Visionary—T

Interpreting these charts provided me the most intense introspective therapy of my entire life. I tease you with all too little information because, of all other personal journeys, there is **none** that can provide you the insights and satisfaction that basic archetypal analysis can!

If you have not yet studied this essential life script, I strongly recommend you do so **now**. Go to Caroline Myss' *Sacred Contracts* or:

Determining Your Archetypes—Caroline Myss

https://www.myss.com/free-resources/sacred-contracts-and-your-archetypes/determining-your-archetypes/

The time has come, the walrus said, to speak of many things! Exploring your archetypes and casting some basic archetypal charts is extraordinarily rewarding.

A Special Meditation

There are many roads to Rome and even more to the soul and spirit. One of my favorites is the Violet Flame, about which I had heard but not studied. I am most grateful to Gail Larmer for giving me permission to use the version she shared with me:

Gail Larmer, 2011 Sacred Heart Connection

The Violet Flame

The violet transmuting flame is one of the most powerful tools in creation for mankind. Working with the violet flame can change wrong conditions and all that is less than perfect, including karma. The violet flame is also called sacred fire and can be compared to a cosmic eraser. The ascended master, Saint Germain, brought forth the teaching of the violet flame to mankind. When invoking the violet flame, ask for the assistance of Saint Germain and his twin flame, Master Lady Portia, along with Archangel Zadkiel, Lady Amethyst, and the violet flame angels.

Before calling on the violet flame, see yourself fully protected within a cocoon of white light and call on the law of forgiveness to cut you free from every person, condition, place, or thing and from every person who owes you something. Ask for the law of forgiveness to balance whatever part that you had in it.

The violet flame will enter through the bottom of your feet and burst into a flame within the body and all around the subtle energies of the body. Visualize the violet flame 9 feet high and 6 feet wide so that you are surrounded completely within a pillar of violet fire.

As you visualize a brilliant, blazing violet fire invoke, the flame with great intention and intensity by saying, **"I am the violet transmuting flame. I ask Saint Germain and Master Lady Portia, Archangel Zadkiel, Lady Amethyst, and the violet flame angels to assist me in transmuting, cleansing, clearing, and releasing all that is not in my highest good at cause, core, and effect, those known**

and unknown from this lifetime and all past lives." Visualize yourself sitting inside this violet flame and continue to say, "**I am the violet flame."** Stay in the violet flame meditation for 5–15 minutes. Using the violet flame daily will bring about great change in your life.

At the end of your violet flame meditation, visualize your physical body being filled with the beautiful pink light of unconditional love and place yourself in a cocoon of pink light. Give thanks and send gratitude to all of the divine beings who assisted with this process.

> "The violet flame is the activity of divine love which consumes or transmutes. It is that rate of vibration. The violet flame is divine alchemy. It cleanses the force fields of the electrons composing the atom which produces a change in vibratory action and results in divine alchemy. The use of the violet flame will change vibratory rates and through transmutation bring about transformation. It is an action of mercy and compassion.
>
> A.D.K. Luk
> *Law of Life Book I*
> Saint Germain

Astrology as a Personality Assessment Tool

I was born at 3:38 a.m. in Columbia, SC on December 4, 1932. This means my sun sign (conscious direction and life focus) is Sagittarius—a fire sign which indicates great stamina and a love of physical activity, outgoing, enthusiastic, and above all bluntly *foot in mouth disease!!* Highly spiritual, confident, philosophical, curious, playful.

My moon, (which influences emotions) is in Pisces, which means strongly intuitive and imaginative, compassionate, easily amused, soft-hearted, empathetic. This requires great practice to prevent absorbing the feelings of those around me! I need solitude to recharge.

My North Node (greatest challenge in this life) is in Pisces, needing to trust in the process of life and surrender anxieties to a higher power.

This also means than my South Node is in Virgo, one who has had great success in past lives in being duty-bound and living according to the rules. Incidentally my wife in this life is a Virgo, as are my closest male friend and an office manager for over twenty-five years. Virgo is a very comfortable feeling to me.

Incidentally it is not uncommon to have the North Node in either your Sun, Moon or Ascendant sign—a double whammy influence!

My ascendant or rising sign is Libra, above all (appreciating fairness and justice), *showing my first natural reaction to new people and situations.* I can be persuasive. Marriage is tremendously significant. I spent the last year before marriage dating at least forty individuals, looking for the perfect mate. Fortunately, that was the most important decision of my life!! My ruling planet of Libra, Venus, is in Scorpio, indicating a strong depth of desire and feeling. Fortunately, this provides me a strong creative force, which has been used for love, healing, and creativity.

Incidentally if either parent's sun sign is in one of your four critical ones, that indicates a very strong connection. My father was Sagittarian and my mother was Pisces.

I strongly advise you to have a chart done. Then you can go to the Internet and search for:

- Meaning of Sun in (which of the 12 signs)
- Meaning of moon in (which of the 12 signs)
- Meaning of ascendant in (which of the 12 signs). Also look up where your ascendant's ruling planet is!
- Meaning of North Node in (which of the 12 signs)

Study these personality influences to assist you in working to optimize all that you **chose** in coming to this life!!! And how to work on your karma!!

A.R.E. PRESS

EDGAR CAYCE'S A.R.E.

Who Was Edgar Cayce?
Twentieth Century Psychic and Medical Clairvoyant

Edgar Cayce (pronounced Kay-Cee, 1877-1945) has been called the "sleeping prophet," the "father of holistic medicine," and the most-documented psychic of the 20th century. For more than 40 years of his adult life, Cayce gave psychic "readings" to thousands of seekers while in an unconscious state, diagnosing illnesses and revealing lives lived in the past and prophecies yet to come. But who, exactly, was Edgar Cayce?

Cayce was born on a farm in Hopkinsville, Kentucky, in 1877, and his psychic abilities began to appear as early as his childhood. He was able to see and talk to his late grandfather's spirit, and often played with "imaginary friends" whom he said were spirits on the other side. He also displayed an uncanny ability to memorize the pages of a book simply by sleeping on it. These gifts labeled the young Cayce as strange, but all Cayce really wanted was to help others, especially children.

Later in life, Cayce would find that he had the ability to put himself into a sleep-like state by lying down on a couch, closing his eyes, and folding his hands over his stomach. In this state of relaxation and meditation, he was able to place his mind in contact with all time and space—the universal consciousness, also known as the super-conscious mind. From there, he could respond to questions as broad as, "What are the secrets of the universe?" and "What is my purpose in life?" to as specific as, "What can I do to help my arthritis?" and "How were the pyramids of Egypt built?" His responses to these questions came to be called "readings," and their insights offer practical help and advice to individuals even today.

The majority of Edgar Cayce's readings deal with holistic health and the treatment of illness. Yet, although best known for this material, the sleeping Cayce did not seem to be limited to concerns about the physical body. In fact, in their entirety, the readings discuss an astonishing 10,000 different topics. This vast array of subject matter can be narrowed down into a smaller group of topics that, when compiled together, deal with the following five categories: (1) Health-Related Information; (2) Philosophy and Reincarnation; (3) Dreams and Dream Interpretation; (4) ESP and Psychic Phenomena; and (5) Spiritual Growth, Meditation, and Prayer.

Learn more at EdgarCayce.org.

What Is A.R.E.?

Edgar Cayce founded the non-profit Association for Research and Enlightenment (A.R.E.) in 1931, to explore spirituality, holistic health, intuition, dream interpretation, psychic development, reincarnation, and ancient mysteries—all subjects that frequently came up in the more than 14,000 documented psychic readings given by Cayce.

The Mission of the A.R.E. is to help people transform their lives for the better, through research, education, and application of core concepts found in the Edgar Cayce readings and kindred materials that seek to manifest the love of God and all people and promote the purposefulness of life, the oneness of God, the spiritual nature of humankind, and the connection of body, mind, and spirit.

With an international headquarters in Virginia Beach, Va., a regional headquarters in Houston, regional representatives throughout the U.S., Edgar Cayce Centers in more than thirty countries, and individual members in more than seventy countries, the A.R.E. community is a global network of individuals.

A.R.E. conferences, international tours, camps for children and adults, regional activities, and study groups allow like-minded people to gather for educational and fellowship opportunities worldwide.

A.R.E. offers membership benefits and services that include a quarterly body-mind-spirit member magazine, Venture Inward, a member newsletter covering the major topics of the readings, and access to the entire set of readings in an exclusive online database.

Learn more at EdgarCayce.org.

EDGARCAYCE.ORG